A primer of emergency imaging

Acute CT:
A primer of emergency imaging

Saeed Mirsadraee MD PhD MRCS FRCR
Specialist Registrar in Clinical Radiology,
Leeds Teaching Hospitals, Leeds, UK

Kshitij Mankad MBBS MRCP FRCR
Specialist Registrar in Clinical Radiology,
Leeds Teaching Hospitals, Leeds, UK

Alan Chalmers MBChB MRCP FRCR
Consultant Radiologist,
Leeds Teaching Hospitals, Leeds, UK

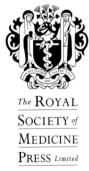

The ROYAL
SOCIETY *of*
MEDICINE
PRESS *Limited*

© 2010 Royal Society of Medicine Press Ltd

Published by the Royal Society of Medicine Press Ltd
1 Wimpole Street, London W1G 0AE, UK
Tel: +44 (0)20 7290 2921
Fax: +44 (0)20 7290 2929
E-mail: publishing@rsm.ac.uk
Website: www.rsmpress.co.uk

British Library Cataloguing in Publication Data
A catalogue record for this book is available from the British Library

ISBN 978-1-85315-742-4

Distribution in Europe and Rest of World:
Marston Book Services Ltd
PO Box 269
Abingdon
Oxon OX14 4YN, UK
Tel: +44 (0)1235 465500
Fax: +44 (0)1235 465555
Email: direct.order@marston.co.uk

Distribution in the USA and Canada:
Royal Society of Medicine Press Ltd
c/o BookMasters, Inc.
30 Amberwood Parkway
Ashland, Ohio 44805, USA

Tel: +1 800 247 6553/ +1 800 266 5564
Fax: +1 419 281 6883
Email: order@bookmasters.com

Distribution in Australia and New Zealand:
Elsevier Australia
30-52 Smidmore Street
Marrikville NSW 2204, Australia
Tel: +61 2 9349 5811
Fax: +61 2 9349 5911
Email: service@elsevier.com.au

Typeset by Phoenix Photosetting, Chatham, Kent, UK
Printed and bound by Bell & Bain Ltd, Glasgow, UK

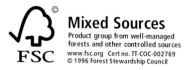

Mixed Sources
Product group from well-managed
forests and other controlled sources
www.fsc.org Cert no. TT-COC-002769
© 1996 Forest Stewardship Council

Contents

Contributing authors

Musculoskeletal trauma

Dr Dominic Baron MBBS BSc(Hons) FRCR
Consultant Musculoskeletal Radiologist, Leeds Teaching Hospitals, Leeds, UK

Neuroradiology and trauma

Dr Jeremy MacMullen-Price, MBChB, MRCP, FRCR
Consultant Neuro-radiologist, Leeds General Infirmary, Leeds, UK

Paediatric radiology and trauma

Dr Leonard Petrus MD
Visiting Assistant Professor of Radiology, Department of Radiological Sciences David Geffen School of Medicine at UCLA Los Angeles, California, USA

Adrienne C Bean MD
Board Certified Paediatrician and Resident of Radiology, Department of Radiology, UCLA Medical Center, Los Angeles, CA, USA

Cardiac and vascular radiology and trauma

David J Tuite MB FFRRCSI
Senior Lecturer, University College Cork School of Medicine, Consultant Radiologist, Cork University Hospital, Cork, Ireland

James C Carr MD MRCPI FFRRCSI FRCR
Associate Professor, Director, Cardiovascular Imaging, Northwestern University Medical School, Department of Radiology, Chicago, IL, USA

1 Introduction

The ever-increasing demand for acute out-of-office hours imaging imposes significant challenges for radiology departments. This demand most often impacts on the more junior radiologists who are usually on the front line of any acute service. Increasingly, the mainstay of out-of-hours radiology is computed tomography (CT), which has become fundamental to decision-making and patient management over a wide range of clinical scenarios, from the acute abdomen to polytrauma. The aim of this book is to provide junior radiologists with a concise overview of the commoner out-of-hours imaging situations they may be faced with. We will describe the expected CT signs for each condition, and emphasize potential pitfalls that might be encountered. Apart from the paediatric and vascular chapters, the protocols described, and the reasoning behind them, reflect current radiological practice in the Leeds Teaching Hospitals NHS Trust, UK. We aim to deliver a consistency in approach to each topic that hopefully will enable the reader to glean quickly the key information needed when dealing with the range of acute events they might meet in routine practice.

Referral practices for acute radiology will vary widely from institution to institution, and will range from a discussion as to the most appropriate examination to a demand for a test with no clinicoradiological liaison. We consider an out-of-hours request should be a two-way scenario that always benefits from discussion between the referrer and the radiologist. The radiologist very much depends on the quality of the clinical information offered, which is fundamental to both choice of investigation and the subsequent interpretation of the images. For the clinician, an understanding of the benefits and the limitations of each imaging technique will help in discussions with the on-call radiologist. We aim to concentrate on the role of acute CT and hope that clinical colleagues will find the content of value in helping them understand the strengths and weaknesses of CT, why we choose certain protocols, and how likely it is that a request for an acute CT will help them manage their patient more effectively. In Chapter 2 we will discuss the basics of CT scanning, and clarify variations in technique and discuss what these mean for clinician and patient. Subsequent sections will then deal with the commoner acute pathologies that might lead to a request for CT.

2 CT Techniques

Multidetector computed tomography

Major advances in CT technology have occurred during the last decade. The majority of systems currently in service for acute CT use multidetector technology. A detailed review of multidetector CT (MDCT) is beyond the scope of this book and there are numerous reviews readily available should the reader require additional background information. For practical purposes, these systems are significantly faster and inherently more flexible than previous generations of scanners. Multidetector systems differ from previous spiral or helical scanners in the number of detector rings used and the significantly increased speed of detector rotation. Early MDCT systems used 4 or 8 detector technology, whereas at the time of writing, 64 detector systems are the norm for general-purpose CT. With 16–64 detector systems, isotropic voxels are generated, which means high-resolution images are no longer restricted to the traditional axial plane but can be reconstructed in axial, coronal, sagittal and off-centre options without any increased radiation penalty to the patient. Current system speeds are illustrated by the 0.33-seconds gantry rotations now standard with 64 detector scanners.

Flexibility in slice thickness selection is a further advantage of MDCT. With spiral or helical CT, slice thickness was fixed and had to be selected before image acquisition, whereas with MDCT, the optimum slice thickness for the presenting clinical problem can be selected after the initial data acquisition. Although theoretically 1 mm slices reconstructed at 1 mm intervals can be chosen, these are inherently noisy images unless significantly higher radiation exposures are used. Producing vast numbers of images in most acute situations is of no benefit to the patient, the reading radiologist or the departmental archive. Averaging the thin section source data allows the choice of a reconstructed slice thickness of some 2.5–5 mm, which is a practical compromise between diagnostic image quality and the radiation dose delivered to the patient for most body imaging.

PACS (picture archiving and communication systems)

The advent of MDCT brought with it the need for radiology departments to adapt to the demands of dealing with an ever-increasing volume of imaging datasets, as well as providing a means of rapidly accessible image review and data manipulation. PACS provides such functionality, and these systems are rapidly replacing conventional hard-copy film reading and scanner-based workstations in many radiology departments. PACS also provides remote and simultaneous access to current and stored imaging data, enabling images to be reviewed by clinicians in the ward, clinic or operating theatre environments, as well as in the radiology department.

Contrast agents used in acute CT

Oral contrast

Conventional CT studies of the abdomen and pelvis routinely use oral contrast to optimize the demonstration of the gastrointestinal tract and aid discrimination between fluid lying within the bowel and fluid located in an extra-enteric position. For acute CT, there are options regarding both the use and type of oral contrast chosen, that are largely determined by the clinical problem under investigation. Oral contrast agents can be considered in two broad groups, namely positive contrast and neutral contrast agents.

Positive contrast agents

These are either iodine based or dilute barium based, and the choice of iodine-based product varies from centre to centre. **Gastrografin** (Bracco; diatrizoate meglumine and diatrizoate sodium solution) is widely used in the UK, but has the disadvantage of being rather unpalatable, as well as having the tendency to produce problematic diarrhoea as a side effect. Low osmolar agents such as **iohexol** (omnipaque; GE Healthcare) offer a more palatable alternative with the added advantages of being poorly absorbed from the gastrointestinal tract and safer to use should aspiration occur.

Dilute barium preparations offer an alternative, such as **E-Z-CAT** (Bracco), a 2.0% w/w preparation that provides comparable opacification of bowel loops to iodine-based products without any associated diarrhoea or nausea.

Positive contrast agents have the advantage when it comes to differentiating between intra-enteric content and an extra-enteric collection, which is important for the radiologist trying to distinguish between what might be an abscess and what might be normal bowel content.

Neutral contrast agents

Water is the commonest, cheapest and most readily available neutral agent used, but it is not the best agent for bowel distension. Alternatives that produce better bowel distension include mannitol solution and commercial products such as VoLumen (Bracco; 0.1% w/v barium sulphate solution). Neutral agents are preferred when the bowel wall or bowel lumen requires particular attention. If a gastrointestinal tract bleed is suspected, neutral agents are chosen as they will enable intraluminal contrast extravasation to be identified, whereas positive agents, due to their high density, may obscure the site of bleeding.

Abdominal CT with no oral contrast

The advent of MDCT with its faster image acquisition and improved image resolution, along with instantly available multiplanar reformatted images, has lessened the need for routine oral contrast. Nevertheless, oral contrast of whatever type would be considered standard practice even in this MDCT-dominated world, particularly in the slim and cachectic patient. There are situations when oral contrast is purposely omitted from the scanning protocol, as described below.

Trauma imaging: In the early days of CT trauma imaging, oral contrast was often withheld because of concerns of potential aspiration. Experience over the years proved this concern to be unfounded and oral contrast became a mandatory requirement for trauma imaging in most trauma centres. The arrival of MDCT has reversed this practice with many units now choosing to omit oral contrast from their standard polytrauma protocols. This change in practice means trauma patients progress more speedily from their initial clinical evaluation and then through CT compared to the era when oral contrast was considered a prerequisite. While all would accept that CT units are not the safest environment for the critically ill, the major advances in scanner speeds, along with the removal of delays caused by an insistence on oral contrast ingestion, has led to an increased clinical acceptance that some unstable patients benefit from a triage CT study on their way to the operating theatre. The traditional teaching reference to CT scanners being the 'doughnut of death' is gradually being replaced by an understanding of the benefits trauma CT can provide both for the trauma surgeon and the interventional radiologist. At the time of writing, the role of CT in the unstable patient remains controversial, and will be discussed again in the Chapter 3.

An exception to the above practice is the patient who presents with penetrating trauma. In this circumstance, many trauma centres advocate the use of both oral and colonic contrast to maximize the detection of bowel injury.

Suspected bowel obstruction: This subject will be discussed in more detail in the Chapter 4, but as a rule, there is no need to give oral contrast to a patient with a high probability of small or large bowel obstruction. The patient will be vomiting and in no mood to consume large quantities of oral contrast. The obstructed small and large bowel will contain plentiful fluid content that provides ideal neutral contrast for CT diagnosis without the need for further contrast ingestion. In the specific situation of potential *subacute* small bowel obstruction, there is an argument for giving oral contrast. If delayed images show contrast in the colon, high-grade obstruction is excluded, giving an opportunity for more conservative management.

Suspected perforation: Departments vary in their approach to this problem, with some giving and others withholding oral contrast. Leakage of low osmolar agents into the peritoneal cavity results in no detrimental effects and identifying extra-luminal oral contrast can be of diagnostic benefit.

Renal stone disease: If the problem posed is solely the need to confirm the presence or absence of renal stone disease, oral contrast is not a requirement for the study.

Rule out acute appendicitis: Some centres favour a study without the use of oral or intravenous contrast. These examinations tend to be targeted at the right iliac fossa rather than being part of a global survey of the whole abdomen and pelvis. Such focused examinations have their supporters and their detractors, and are better suited to the more obese than cachectic patient.

How much oral contrast should be given?

A pragmatic approach is always needed to balance what is reasonable and practicable with what would represent the perfect study. Speed is often of the essence in acute imaging and an unreasonable study delay to optimize bowel opacification is not recommended. As a general guide, about a litre of contrast is required to demonstrate the abdominal and pelvic small bowel loops. However, the ingestion of such a volume may not be realistic and in some clinical circumstances, reducing the contrast volume to 500 ml will at least opacify the upper abdominal small bowel loops, helping in the assessment of upper gastrointestinal pathology involving the pancreas and the duodenal sweep. For the patient who cannot tolerate drinking this volume of fluid, delivery via a nasogastric tube offers an alternative approach.

Oral contrast allergy

This is extremely rare but if there is a compelling history of prior severe contrast allergy, selecting a barium-based contrast agent rather than an iodine-based preparation makes practical sense.

Intravenous contrast agents

When do we use them? Intravenous contrast is essential for certain acute CT studies, such as the detection of pulmonary embolic disease, the diagnosis of bowel ischaemia and the demonstration of pancreatic parenchymal necrosis. Intravenous contrast is not required for the detection of renal stone disease and as discussed, is optional in other situations such as acute appendicitis. However, whether intravenous contrast is given or withheld may be determined by the patient's renal status or any accompanying history of prior contrast allergy or severe atopy.

Renal function and the use of intravenous contrast

Patients with disordered renal function who are exposed to intravenous contrast are at increased risk of developing the complication of contrast-induced nephropathy. Other clinical states when intravenous contrast is associated with a higher risk of complication include diabetes, multiple myeloma, poor cardiac function, and the use of drugs that are known to be nephrotoxic, such as aminoglycosides.

Assessment of renal function prior to contrast-enhanced CT varies from centre to centre. Ignoring a patient's renal function is not recommended as contrast-induced nephropathy is a cause of significant morbidity. The simplest option, used by many departments, is to evaluate the **serum creatinine**. If the serum creatinine is elevated – in our department in excess of 150 μmol/L – a decision has to be made whether greater potential harm than good may result from the use of intravenous contrast. Other centres prefer to rely on the **glomerular filtration rate** as a more accurate determinant of a patient's renal status. As well as serum creatinine, this method will factor in variations due to body weight, age, sex and ethnic background.

Several options are open to the radiologist when faced with a patient who has known renal function impairment:

1. The level of risk can be diminished with prior and post study hydration.
2. Smaller volumes of contrast can be used.
3. Contrast agents with lower iodine concentrations are preferred.
4. Select an iso-osmolar agent such as Visipaque (Iodixanol; GE Healthcare) that has a proven benefit over conventional low osmolar agents when renal function is a problem.

(Ionic contrast agents are no longer used for contrast-enhanced CT.)

Venous access

An anticubital fossa vein is the preferred site for venous cannulation. Small back of hand veins should only be used if no alternative is available and the use of foot veins is an interpretative complication too many. Contrast is generally delivered via a power injector. In adult patients, MDCT protocols will typically use about 100–150 ml of contrast delivered at a rate of 3 ml/s for conventional abdominal imaging, increasing to 4–5 ml/s for studies where vascular assessment is paramount.

The use of central lines for contrast delivery is controversial and each department will have its own policy with regard to whether or not these are used. Hand injection rather than power injector contrast delivery is preferred, and power injectors should not be used with conventional PICC (peripherally inserted central catheter) lines. Recently, PICC lines have been developed which are power injector friendly – 'Power PICCs'. These are always clearly labelled as being injector friendly. If in any doubt, do *not* use them.

Phases of contrast delivery

MDCT allows the radiologist to modify the examination to best answer specific clinical questions. One method of achieving this is to consider whether a single phase study will suffice or whether multiple phases are required to optimize diagnosis. For the purpose of acute CT, contrast delivery can be considered in three specific 'time from injection' phases, namely arterial, portal venous and delayed phases, with the flexibility of MDCT enabling single or multiple phases to be incorporated into the chosen scanning protocol. It should be remembered that *any increase in the number of phases will result in an increase in the radiation dose.* The radiologist must balance what represents an appropriate protocol to provide a diagnosis with what might result in an excessive and inappropriate radiation dose to the patient.

Standard survey CT protocols of the abdomen and pelvis are timed to cover the liver at the optimum time to detect focal lesions, produce uniform parenchymal enhancement of the solid organs, and optimize demonstration of the portal and hepatic venous anatomy. This is known as the **portal venous phase** and occurs some 50–60 s after the onset of contrast delivery, assuming no adverse factors such as poor venous access or compromised cardiac function.

Arterial phase imaging: This is performed to optimally demonstrate the arterial vascular anatomy, and takes place approximately 20–25 s post onset of contrast injection. The patient's circulatory function will have a major impact on start of scan timings, but the guess work of judging when to scan has largely been removed from modern CT practice with the use of computer programs which evaluate the rate of early aortic contrast enhancement after a small tracking contrast bolus is injected. The exact time to maximize arterial contrast enhancement can then be built into the scan protocol. Arterial enhancement can also be improved by the use of a saline flush 'chaser', which is injected after the contrast has been delivered. This clears any contrast which might pool in the cannulated and delivery veins, and in so doing reduces streak artefact in vessels such as the superior vena cava, which can be problematic during chest imaging.

Delayed phase imaging: This is most commonly used in trauma imaging. When an injury to the renal tract is shown on the portal venous phase series, a delayed acquisition after 5–10 min can be invaluable for demonstrating opacified urine extravasating from the renal collecting system or ureter. A further use for delayed phase CT is to distinguish between a traumatic pseudoaneurysm or arteriovenous malformation and active contrast extravasation from an injured solid organ or vessel. A contained vascular injury will display contrast washout with time comparable to an adjacent intact vessel. A focus of active contrast extravasation will maintain or increase its density with time. In this circumstance, the delayed series is performed immediately following review of the portal venous phase acquisition.

Biphasic or triphasic imaging: The speed of data acquisition with MDCT allows the acquisition of multiple contrast phases without hardware restrictions, such as problematic tube cooling, a feature of earlier generations of scanners. Biphasic imaging will typically include both arterial and portal venous phases, whereas triple phase studies will include either an initial unenhanced series or a delayed acquisition along with arterial and portal venous acquisitions.

Interstitial phase imaging: This is specific to pancreatic imaging where it confers a theoretical advantage for assessing pancreatic parenchymal enhancement and deciding whether necrosis is present during the evaluation of acute pancreatitis. The interstitial phase occurs some 35–40 s after onset of injection.

Intravenous contrast reactions

Recording a history of prior contrast reaction or a history of severe atopy is part of a CT radiographer's pre-study responsibilities, and when such a history is established, a decision is required as to whether intravenous contrast is needed for that particular clinical problem. Each radiology department will have protocols to deal with contrast reactions and also to provide a robust system of recording such events to prevent future problems for the patient concerned. In the event of a reaction, the patient must be made fully aware of what has happened and counselled regarding the future use of intravenous contrast.

A detailed discussion of contrast reactions and their treatment is outside the scope of this book and the reader is referred to the articles by Namasivayam et al and Wang referenced at the end of this chapter. A quick reference to the treatment of this condition is given in the Appendix.

- **Severe contrast reactions** to iodinated contrast using low osmolar or iso-osmolar agents are extremely rare (<0.05%). These include laryngeal oedema and cardiopulmonary arrest, and will require immediate treatment often with the assistance of the emergency crash team. Death is vanishingly rare with a reported incidence of 1 in 1 000 000.
- **Intermediate severity reactions** such as mild bronchospasm or urticarial rash usually require intervention with bronchodilators and antihistamines, respectively.
- **Mild reactions** include nausea, vomiting and pruritis, and typically settle with minimal supportive care.
- **Delayed reactions** are a recognized complication and can occur hours to days after the event. Fortunately, these are almost exclusively restricted to skin rashes.

Premedication regimens for patients with a prior history of contrast reaction are practised with varying enthusiasm from department to department. These are unlikely to factor in the acute CT situation and, it should be remembered, will reduce but not eliminate the risk of further reaction. A reasonable approach for acute CT is that if in doubt, do *not* give contrast. If intravenous contrast is a necessity for diagnosis in a clinically worrisome situation, a clinicoradiological decision is required to evaluate risk of harm versus diagnostic benefit. In the UK, most CT departments do not routinely obtain consent for intravenous contrast. In the USA, such consent is usually considered mandatory.

Patients on metformin

Metformin hydrochloride (glucophage) is a recognized albeit rare cause of lactic acidosis in patients receiving intravenous contrast. Although the incidence of this complication is very low, current UK practice dictates that due caution is required when intravenous contrast is given to a patient on metformin medication. Metformin should be stopped for 48 hours post study and only restarted when a reassessment of renal function shows no abnormality.

Rectal contrast

The only routine use for rectal contrast in acute CT is the evaluation of penetrating trauma. In this specific circumstance, opacification of the large bowel will aid the detection of colonic injury and may show extra-enteric contrast, confirming bowel penetration. A litre of 3% contrast is delivered by drip infusion gravity feed via a rectal catheter. The catheter is removed following gravity drainage of contrast at the end of the study.

Bladder contrast

This is another trauma related technique. The preferred method of confirming or excluding bladder injury is to perform a CT cystogram after the initial polytrauma study, the indication for this study being the demonstration of pelvic fractures and concern of associated bladder injury. The technique involves the delivery of 500 ml of 3% iodinated contrast under gravity feed or gentle hand injection via a urinary catheter. Catheter placement should be the responsibility of the trauma clinician. CT cystography is superior to the alternative option of performing delayed imaging once opacified urine has reached the urinary bladder. CT cystography will confirm the diagnosis of intraperitoneal and extraperitoneal extravasation with a diagnostic accuracy approaching 100%.

Radiation issues

It is the responsibility of the supervising radiologist to prevent excessive or inappropriate use of ionizing radiation. As has been well publicised in the medical and popular press, the explosion in demand for CT scanning has resulted in CT being responsible for the major proportion of radiation delivered to the general population via medical imaging. By way of illustration, in 1980 some three million CT examinations were performed in the USA, contrasting with some 62 million in 2006. The success of MDCT has further fuelled this explosion with its benefits leading to increased use in a variety of areas, such as vascular and cardiac imaging and CT colonography.

As a guide for the non-radiologist reader, the Table 2.1 gives an indication of the radiation doses involved.

In the young and the pregnant, alternative imaging options such as ultrasound and magnetic resonance (MR), which avoid ionizing radiation, should always be explored in the first instance. The preferred initial investigation for right upper quadrant pain should always be ultrasound

Table 2.1: Illustrative radiation doses

Investigation	Radiation dose (mSv)
CXR	0.1
Abdominal CT	5.3
Chest CT	5.8
Chest, abdo and pelvic CT	9.9

rather than CT, and similarly in the evaluation of pelvic or right iliac fossa pain in a young female, ultrasound should be the initial test. MR can be an invaluable diagnostic tool for a variety of acute abdominal pathologies in the pregnant patient, including renal tract compromise secondary to stone disease, acute appendicitis and bowel obstruction. Despite its benefits, MR may not be readily available as an out-of-hours option for general body imaging.

The radiation dose to a patient depends on a number of variables, including the volume of anatomy scanned, the patient's physical build, the type and number of scan phases, and the overall image quality required. Modern CT systems incorporate a number of dose-reducing features, one of the commoner being an auto milliampere setting. This allows the scanner to adjust the radiation dose delivered to anatomical areas which display inherent density differences, such as chest and abdominal cavities, as well as taking account of differing body habitus. This dose reduction does not affect the resultant image quality.

CT and the pregnant patient

Whenever possible, avoiding ionizing radiation in the pregnant patient is sound practice, particularly in the first trimester. Nevertheless, recent studies of estimated foetal doses support the conclusion that the risks are minimal and that the potential benefits of significant diagnostic information should not be withheld from the pregnant patient. It remains essential that when CT is used in pregnancy, the protocol used must minimize the radiation dose delivered.

It is also sensible practice to avoid intravenous contrast in pregnancy unless essential for diagnosis. When necessary, non-ionic contrast is considered safe to use with no proven adverse effects on the neonatal thyroid.

CT and children

Young growing children are potentially at increased risk from ionizing radiation and as such, careful consideration must be given when requesting X-ray studies, as well as the use of alternative imaging techniques such as ultrasound and MRI. While the CT protocol has to be modified to reduce radiation dose, at the same time diagnostic quality must be maintained to avoid unnecessary repeat examinations.

Recommended reading

Bone JM. Multidetector CT: opportunities, challenges and concerns associated with 64 or more detector systems. *Radiology* 2006:**241**:334–7.

McCollough CH, Schueler BA, Atwell TD, et al. Radiation exposure and pregnancy: when should we be concerned? *Radiographics* 2007;**27**: 909–18.

Namasivayam S, Kalra MK, Torres WE, Small WC. Adverse reaction to intravenous iodinated contrast media; a primer for radiologists. *Emerg Radiol* 2006;**12**:210–15.

Wang CL. Frequency, outcome and appropriateness of treatment of non ionic contrast media reactions. *AJR Am J Roentgenol* 2008;**191**:409–15.

3 Trauma

Overview

Trauma refers to injuries caused by external force or violence. These range from minor to major, obvious to occult and single injury to multi-focal. This can make imaging difficult to target correctly. Very minor peripheral trauma can often be adequately assessed by clinical examination alone, whereas a polytrauma victim will require a full body CT.

The key to targeting this correctly is to consider the mechanism involved in combination with the clinical findings. Patients tend to then fall into three definite categories:

1. Low energy mechanism with no clinical concern for any significant injury. Patient can be assessed and treated on clinical grounds alone.
2. Low energy mechanism with significant clinical concern that requires imaging, often by plain radiographs initially.
3. High-energy mechanism which requires imaging.

What constitutes a high-energy mechanism? A significant amount of research has been done on this with regards to cervical spine trauma and the following are generally regarded as 'high-energy' mechanisms:

- Road traffic accident at over 35 mph combined impact.
- Pedestrian struck by car.
- Motorcycle accident.
- Fall from > 3 m.
- Crash with death at scene.
- Polytrauma.
- Neurological signs or symptoms referred to cervical spine (c-spine).
- Significant closed head injury.

Although these criteria are aimed at cervical spine imaging, they also hold up for all trauma. This is because high-energy mechanisms tend to cause multiple injuries rather than affect areas in isolation.

As already stated, when investigating a high-energy mechanism the current trend is to perform whole body CT scanning, now that multislice technology is firmly established. This is very useful in terms of fully evaluating the patient, but the question often raised is whether the radiation dose incurred is justifiable.

The simple answer to this is that all investigations using ionizing radiation have to be justified under the radiation regulation acts. In the context of a high-energy accident where there is a high risk of injury, the consequences of missing a life-threatening injury far surpass the risk of the diagnostic radiation. Put another way, the patient must survive their major trauma with whatever injuries they have acquired to live long enough to develop any cancers secondary to the radiation dose.

This does not mean that dose should be ignored. Care must be taken to always keep the dose to the minimum required to generate diagnostic data. The newer scanners have numerous hardware and software options that assist with this and it is essential to ensure that these are optimized to ensure compliance with ALARA (As Low As Reasonably Achievable).

Adult musculoskeletal trauma

Cervical spine

Summary

Protocol: Thin slice (1 mm) volume acquisition through the whole cervical spine down to the bottom of T1 and preferably T4 with sagittal and coronal reformats. This can be part of a full polytrauma study.

What to look for: Loss of alignment in any plane, fractures at any level and in any plane. Do not forget the occipital condyles and skull base.

Report: Describe all injuries seen and their potential for instability, although this can only be implied from a static study. A normal CT does not fully clear the cervical spine which requires a combination of clinical and radiological findings.

Cervical spine injuries create a significant workload for the Accident & Emergency (A&E) Department. The majority of patients will turn out to have nothing more than a soft tissue injury, but the potential for missing a serious injury makes the assessment of spinal trauma one of the most stressful problems emergency clinicians face.

As only a small percentage of these patients will turn out to have a significant injury, it is inappropriate to image everyone. The key to good management of these patients is a high-quality clinical history and examination that allows patients to be stratified into groups to facilitate treatment and investigation. The most widely used triaging tool is the Canadian c-spine rules. Patients are defined as high or low risk as below:

- *High-risk factors*:
  - ☐ Age > 65 years.
  - ☐ Dangerous mechanism.
  - ☐ Paraesthesia in extremities.
- *Low-risk factors*:
  - ☐ Simple rear end shunt.
  - ☐ Sitting position in A&E.
  - ☐ Delayed onset of neck pain.
  - ☐ Absence of midline c-spine tenderness.

High-risk patients require imaging and are discussed later. Patients fulfilling the low-risk criteria do not require initial imaging but do require careful clinical examination. If they are able to actively rotate their neck 45° to the left and right, they are cleared clinically and require no imaging. If they cannot be cleared at this point, they are imaged by the three-view standard c-spine radiographic series. If this series is equivocal or there is persisting clinical concern for an injury, further imaging is required. Where there is concern for bony injury, CT is indicated. The more problematic patients are those for whom concern is for a purely soft tissue/ligamentous injury.

In the low-risk group, flexion/extension studies are often advocated. In the conscious patient these may be useful at 7–10 days, when muscle spasm has settled, but they have no proven value at the initial presentation. A pragmatic approach favoured by many where there is concern for a soft tissue injury in a low-risk patient with no other risk factors (e.g. neurology), is to fit the patient with a hard collar and ask them to re-attend in 7–10 days for supervised flexion/extension views. Most patients then self-select and do not re-attend or take off the collar. Any patients still symptomatic while wearing their collar will require supervised flexion/extension views.

Where there are other concerns, such as abnormal neurology, acute MRI is the favoured approach.

Indications for CT c-spine

The high-risk factors described above give the patient about a 10% chance of a c-spine fracture. The key to identifying all of these is that the energy involved must be far greater than that for the usual, relatively minor bumps.

In addition, all motorcycle crashes and patients who have failed to be cleared by the Canadian c-spine pathway should undergo CT of the whole spine as the next step.

Why CT whole c-spine?

Plain radiographs are poor in upper c-spine with a substantive miss rate (up to 39%).

The cervicothoracic junction is almost always inadequately demonstrated on plain radiographs in polytrauma cases. In addition, there is an even distribution of injuries throughout the c-spine with multilevel injuries being well described.

Protocol and technique

Contrast enhancement: No contrast enhancement is indicated, unless the vertebral and carotid vessels are being screened at the same time.

Slice collimation: The whole of the cervical spine from the occiput to the bottom of T4 should be included. This should be in 1 mm sections with sagittal and coronal reformats.

Algorithm and windowing: A bone algorithm with standard bone windows is sufficient.

What to look for on CT

- It is essential to carefully review the whole cervical spine, including the skull base on axial, sagittal and coronal reformats. Fractures may only show up as linear breaks in the cortices and do not have to be significantly displaced. These should not be confused with vascular markings. The latter only appear on one to two slices and lie in typical locations. The other common error is to mistake normal variants for fractures. These have well-demarcated sclerotic edges and again occur in typical locations.
- Particular attention should be given to the upper cervical spine and occipital condyles where fractures can be very subtle and all three reformats are often needed to make the diagnosis (C1 fracture). When a fracture is detected, it is essential to check adjacent levels as there is a high incidence of contiguous fractures (Fig. 3.1).
- Upper cervical injuries include Jefferson fractures, Hangman's fractures and Peg fracture. A full description of each of these is outside the remit of this text but they can be very difficult to see on

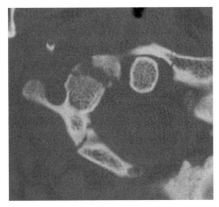

Figure 3.1: C1 ring fracture. Axial image showing multiple fractures of the C1 ring.

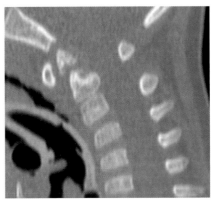

Figure 3.2: Peg fracture. Sagittal reformat showing fracture through the peg with loss of the normal alignment.

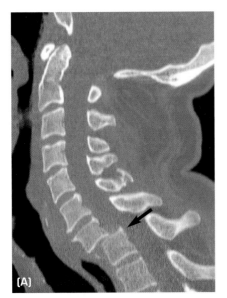

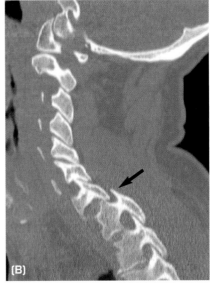

Figure 3.3: Bifacet dislocation. **(A)** Midline sagittal reformat showing the loss of alignment at C7/T1 with approximately 60% anterior slip (arrow). **(B)** Parasagittal reformat demonstrating the anterior dislocation of the C7 inferior articular facet over the T1 superior articular facet (arrow).

plain radiographs. These tend to be more common in the elderly (Fig. 3.2).

■ In the lower cervical spine, flexion, extension and lateral compression injuries predominate. Flexion injuries start with disruption of posterior structures and usually result in widening of the spinous processes and an angular kyphosis. These include facet dislocation, subluxation and perched facets (bifacet dislocation) (Fig. 3.3).

- Extension injuries in contrast start by injuring anterior structures, but often then spring back into a rough normal alignment despite significant soft tissue injuries. Enlargement of the prevertebral soft tissue shadow is more common with these injuries.

- Lateral compression fractures involve the lateral masses and can be very subtle. These facet fractures are not uncommon and subtle loss of alignment on the lateral view is often the only sign of these.

Acute reporting

- All injuries should be carefully described and eponyms avoided. For the junior radiologist, it is unwise to state whether an injury is a flexion/extension or a compression injury, as there are a wide range of patterns described. Leading on from this, although the full extent of the injury should be described, it must be remembered that CT is a static study and stability, or lack of it, can only be implied from the imaging.

- Where a negative study is reported, it is prudent to add the following caveat: 'Please note that this does exclude a pure ligamentous injury'. This will remind the referring clinician that they have to clear the spine based on all findings and not rely purely upon radiology.

- *C-spine clearance:* Does a good quality CT with plain radiographs clear the c-spine? Some centres do adopt this policy, although it remains controversial and not adequately proven. The main concern is for pure ligamentous injuries, particularly in an unconscious patient. Most centres look at the combination of clinical and radiological findings and then clear the c-spine. Where there is ongoing clinical concern or any evidence of neurology, MRI is then indicated.

Thoracic and lumbar spine injuries

Summary

Protocol: Non-contrast enhanced axial dataset (2 mm) with sagittal and coronal reformats. This can be as part of a full polytrauma acquisition.

What to look for: Paravertebral haematoma, posterior column injuries. In particular, look for splaying of the spinous processes and associated intra-abdominal injuries.

Report: The type of injury, as this is prognostic and assists management.

Thoracolumbar spinal injuries have a high incidence in polytrauma, but are often overlooked and are potentially devastating. It is mandatory to actively look for these. There are many classifications used to describe thoracic and lumbar trauma but the simple three-column system by Denis is by far the most useful, both for the reporting radiologist and the surgeon.

Fracture types

It is essential to know the types of injury that occur in this area in order to know what you are looking for. The **column system** splits the spinal anatomy into zones. *The anterior column* extends from the anterior vertebral body cortex to two-thirds of the way back through the body. *The middle column* then extends back to the middle of the spinal canal. *The posterior column* extends posteriorly from this line.

- **Wedge compression fractures:** These are hyperflexion injuries and involve only the anterior column (one column). With these there is disruption to the anterior cortex of the body and usually the superior endplate, but there is no extension to the posterior cortex of the body. These are stable injuries and may also occur in osteoporotic patients with no significant history of trauma.
- **Burst fractures:** These involve both the anterior and middle columns (two columns). The fracture line extends to involve the posterior cortex of the body. This ranges from a minor crack through to a large retropulsed fragment lying in the canal. Burst fractures which only involve the vertebral body are termed incomplete burst fractures and are often stable. Complete burst fracture have a split in the lamina. These are often unstable (Fig. 3.4).

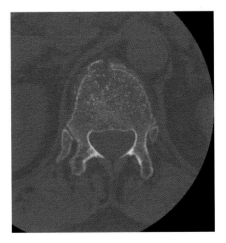

Figure 3.4: Burst fracture. Axial image showing disruption to the concavity of the anterior cortex of the vertebral body consistent with a burst fracture.

■ ***Chance fracture:*** These are hyperflexion injuries and involve all three columns (Fig. 3.5). The fracture line extends across all three columns in a transverse manner and can be purely through bone (body, pedicle and spinous process), purely soft tissue injury (intervertebral disc and interspinous ligaments) or a combination of both. With this fracture combination alignment is maintained in a sagittal and coronal plane. These have a high association with mesenteric, pancreatic and duodenal injuries.

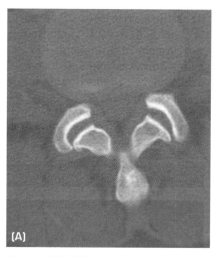
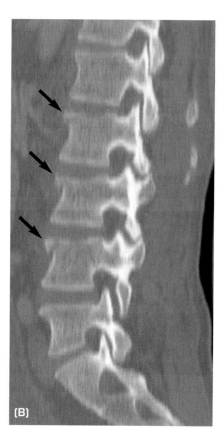

Figure 3.5: Three-column lumbar spine fracture. **(A)** Axial image at the L4/5 level showing widening of both the facet joints. **(B)** Parasagittal reformats confirms the axial abnormality as well as anterior compression injuries to the upper endplates of L2/3/4 (arrows).

■ ***Fracture dislocation:*** These are massive injuries involving all three columns. They are by definition dislocations so, although there is usually marked bony fragmentation, the key to the diagnosis is the loss of alignment of the spine, either in the sagittal or coronal plane (Fig. 3.6).

Protocol and technique

Contrast enhancement: No oral or intravenous contrast is required.

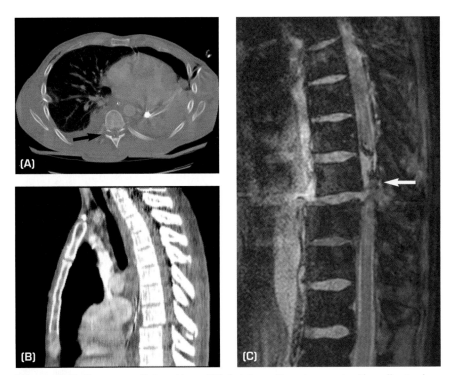

Figure 3.6: Fracture dislocation. (A) Axial section demonstrating diastasis of the facet joints (arrow). Bilateral chest drains in situ with a large left haemopneumothorax. **(B)** Sagittal reformat showing the loss of alignment consistent with a fracture dislocation. **(C)** Sagittal gradient echo MRI demonstrating the fracture dislocation with a transected cord. The arrow points at the susceptibility artefact secondary to haematoma.

Slice collimation: There are three scenarios to cover:

1. ***Polytrauma scan:*** The thoracolumbar spine should be formally evaluated as part of this protocol. A minimum slice thickness of 2.5 mm is necessary with sagittal and coronal reformats. Multislice scanners allow fused 5 mm images to be unfused to generate 2.5 mm images.
2. ***A whole spine protocol:*** A minimum of 2 mm slice thickness should be used for whole spine coverage with sagittal and coronal reformats.
3. ***Fine detail targeted study:*** Where further detail is required, 1 mm slices through the area of interest plus one vertebral body above and below is necessary, again with sagittal and coronal reformats.

Algorithm and windowing: For a dedicated study, a bone algorithm alone is adequate and will keep the dose down. Wide windows for bone are necessary and, where there has been previous surgery, a very wide window will significantly reduce the amount of metalwork artefact.

What to look for on CT

- With all high energy injuries (apart from osteoporotic collapses) other injuries thoraco-lumbar fractures need to be actively excluded. Sternal fractures are associated with both thoracic fractures and aortic injuries.
- Paravertebral haematoma is clearly visible on axial imaging and is a good indirect pointer to spinal fractures. The spinal anatomy needs to be reviewed in all three planes as fractures are often only clearly visible in one plane.
- The posterior cortex of the vertebral body is a key area that requires review in both the axial and sagittal planes. Fractures here can be very subtle with sometimes only a flattening of the normal posterior concavity visible. This is an important finding, as by definition, the injury becomes a two-column fracture.
- Chance fractures may be very obvious but as described, all combinations are possible and sometimes it is only widening of the interspinous gap posteriorly that alerts the reader to the presence of this injury.
- Multilevel injuries are common so that when one injury level is identified, a detailed search for other involved levels should be carried out. Indeed, the *ATLS Manual* states that 50% of spinal fractures have an associated contiguous level fracture and that there is a 10% incidence of non-contiguous spinal fracture. The surgeon, when fixing these, needs to know where the next intact level is located both above and below the main injury level.

Differential diagnosis

The most important factor when assessing spinal injuries is to determine whether the mechanism matches the injury and whether there was sufficient energy involved to produce the injury. If the answer to either of these is no, then it may be that the fracture is pathological; either osteoporotic or tumour related. Osteoporotic compression fractures are often multiple with depression of the endplates and cortical preservation.

With metastases and myeloma, the bone texture tends to be more ill-defined with loss of the cortex. The posterior body cortex is often convex into the spinal canal rather than the usual concavity. Pedicular involvement and significant additional soft tissue are typical findings, often best assessed by MRI.

Interventional aspects

CT can be used to guide biopsy when tumour/infection is suspected.

Acute reporting

- In the acute stage, it is essential to document all the involved levels as well as recording the normal levels to aid surgical planning. At each level, the severity of the injury should be assessed by the three-column system.
- The most important consideration is to carefully look for other injuries. It is essential to remember that these are usually high-energy injuries requiring a full evaluation of the patient for other bony and soft tissue damage is essential.

Facial injuries

Summary

Protocol: Non-contrast thin slice acquisition, coronal views.

What to look for: Pterygoid plates, base of skull, temporomandibular joint (TMJ).

Reporting: Describe the injuries; they usually occur in combinations.

The face has an extremely complex bony anatomy with multiple sinuses. In head trauma the face often acts as a crumple zone and therefore acts to protect the much more important intracranial contents. Bony trauma to this area can be very daunting to interpret as it often results in combination injuries.

Protocol and technique

Contrast enhancement: No contrast enhancement is necessary.

Slice collimation: Thin slice (1 mm) volumetric acquisition from the top of the orbits down to the bottom of the mandible with routine coronal reformats. This may be incorporated into a full polytrauma scan

Algorithm and windowing: A bone algorithm with standard bone windows is sufficient.

What to look for on CT

The pterygoid plates are key to the interpretation of this area. If these are fractured then a LeFort type injury is confirmed; if not, one of the other facial fracture combinations is present. Apart from the bony discontinuity, sinus opacification and air in soft tissues are good indirect signs of these injuries.

■ *Le Fort fractures:* (Fig. 3.7) These were originally described as bilateral symmetrical fractures. These are extremely rare in their pure form and therefore this classification is of little use. A far more valuable classification is to assess each side of the face individually and subdivide the injuries into hemi-LeFort fractures. It is now well recognized that it is possible to have more than one LeFort type injury on each side, and therefore it is possible to have a hemi-LeFort 1/2/3 on one side.

The key to the definition is the presence of a pterygoid plate fracture, which by definition any LeFort-type fracture must have.

☐ **Hemi-LeFort 1:** Fractures of both the lateral and medial walls of the maxillary antrum.
☐ **Hemi-LeFort 2:** Fractures of the lateral wall of the maxillary antrum as well as the orbital floor and medial orbital wall.
☐ **Hemi-LeFort 3:** Fractures of the lateral orbital wall and the medial orbital floor.

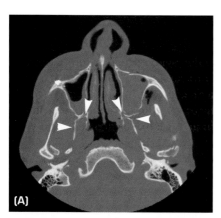

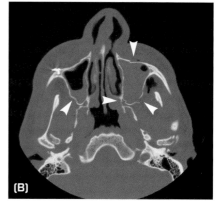

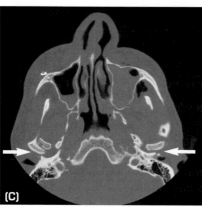

Figure 3.7: LeFort type injury. This case has multiple severe fractures shown on all three axial CT images. **(A)** The arrowheads point to the bilateral pterygoid plate fractures, making this a LeFort type injury. **(B)** The arrowheads highlight the multiple fractures of maxillary antra. **(C)** The arrows point to the bilateral fracture dislocations of the temporomandibular joints.

- *Zygomatico-maxillary complex (ZMC) fractures:* This injury complex used to be termed the tripod fracture. It is now recognized that there are in reality five fractures present. The combination of fractures separates the zygomatic bone leading to a clinically flattened cheekbone. The pterygoid plates are intact but there are fractures to the zygomatic arch, the orbital floor, the lateral orbital wall, the posterolateral and anterolateral walls of the maxillary antrum. Blood in the maxillary antrum is usually present.
- *Naso-orbital ethmoid (NOE) fractures:* These are caused by a direct blow to the nose and can potentially involve the superior sagittal sinus. This mechanism essentially drives the nasal bones back into the ethmoid, leading to fractures of the ethmoid plates, the nasal bones and the frontal bone at the superior orbital rim.
- *Isolated fractures:* Injuries to the medial maxillary antrum, the zygomatic arch, nasal bones and the mandible can all occur in isolation and should be actively excluded. Remember that an injury to the mandible often results in a second mandibular injury as it forms a ring with the temperomandibular joints (TMJs).

Acute reporting

- The key is the pterygoid plates: if they are fractured, it is a LeFort type injury; and if not, the other fracture combinations should be considered.
- Do not forget to look for intracranial/base of skull or cervical spine fractures at the same time as these may be far more important clinically than the facial trauma.
- Be careful to not overlook TMJ dislocations. These will be clearly demonstrated on the axial dataset but are often missed when there are multiple other injuries are present.

Pelvis

Summary

Protocol: Non-contrast thin slice volumetric acquisition, coronal and sagittal views.

What to look for: Active bleeding. The pelvis is a bony ring so it is essential to document all fractures.

Report: Describe the type of injuries and any evidence of active bleeding or associated organ injuries.

The pelvic radiograph still retains its place in the ATLS Primary Survey due to the risk of severe bleeding from a pelvic injury. The pelvic ring is extremely strong and requires a major force to disrupt it. When disruption is identified, it is very important to actively exclude other injury, which is why pelvic fractures are often now scanned as part of a whole body trauma scan. It is essential not to focus solely on the obvious pelvic injury whilst the patient is actively bleeding from a solid organ injury.

It is still common practice for surgeons to immediately put an external fixator on a pelvic fracture. This makes any subsequent vascular intervention awkward. A more pragmatic approach is to look for active bleeding on the initial scan and, if the patient is not haemodynamically stabilized by a simple wrap, then to involve the vascular interventionalists immediately.

Pelvic injuries can be split into pelvic ring injuries and acetabular injuries. With pelvic ring injuries, it is essential to carefully evaluate the whole pelvis as these injuries often present in combination with other areas of focal trauma.

Acetabular fractures can be present in isolation. There are multiple complex classifications which are beyond the remit of this text, but the most commonly used one is the LeTournel and Judet classification.

Protocol and technique

Pelvic imaging is usually performed as part of a polytrauma study (see above). Thin slice volumetric acquisition with coronal views are needed to assess pelvic bones. Where there is a definite fracture, then additional sagittal reformats are indicated.

Contrast enhancement: IV contrast will usually be given as part of a standard polytrauma scan to exclude non-bony injuries.

What to look for on CT

- ***Pelvic ring injuries:*** There are three main groups:
  - ☐ **Anterior compression:** Anteriorly, these classically have pubic symphyseal separation or vertical ramal fractures. Posteriorly, there can be widening of the sacroiliac joints (SIJs) and in very severe cases complete SIJ diastasis. A small percentage have sacral fractures, although these are more common with lateral compression and vertical shear injuries. Anterior compression injuries are potentially haemodynamically unstable injuries, but they usually respond well to a sling which acts to reduce the pelvic volume. If this is unsuccessful, any active bleeding requires the immediate involvement of the vascular interventionalists (Fig. 3.8).

☐ **Lateral compression:** These often have associated acetabular fractures/dislocations. Anteriorly, they tend to be associated with coronally orientated ramal fractures compared with the sagittal pattern seen with anterior compression injuries. Lateral compression injuries do not cause symphyseal diastasis. Posteriorly, they classically result in sacral fractures and in severe cases it is possible to have a sacral fracture on the injured side with a SIJ diastasis on the contralateral side, giving the windswept pelvis appearance. They are often haemodynamically stable as the nature of these injuries is to reduce the pelvic volume that helps tamponade any bleeding points.

☐ **Vertical shear:** These are classically associated with falls and are extremely unstable both mechanically and haemodynamically. The key to the diagnosis of these is either the plain radiograph or the

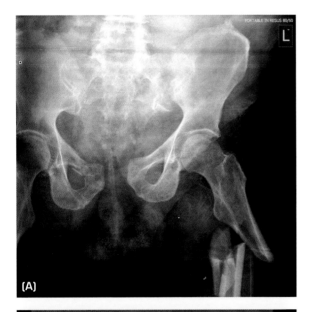

(A)

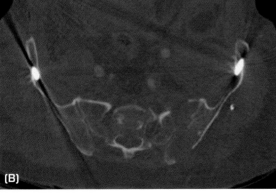

(B)

Figure 3.8: Anterior compression pelvic injury. **(A)** Anteroposterior radiograph shows pubic symphyseal diastasis, fractures to right pubic ramus, disruption to the left sacroiliac joint, and complex fracture upper left femur. **(B)** Axial CT image post pelvic fixation confirms fracture running through the left sacral ala, left sacroiliac joint and left iliac bone.

coronal reformat, where it will become apparent that one of the hemipelvices is cranially displaced (vertical shear).

- *Acetabulum:* There are 20 different types of acetabular fractures described in the literature. These require axial, coronal and sagittal reformats. For the purposes of the acute report, it is sufficient to recognize that there is an injury that requires specialist review. Any injury to the posterior wall/lip of the acetabulum must raise the possibility of a relocated fracture dislocation. As the sciatic nerve lies directly posterior to the acetabulum it is at high risk of injury and this possibility should be raised with the clinicians.

- *Bladder/urethral injuries:* There is a high incidence of injury to these structures with pelvic fractures, and if a catheter is in situ, a CT cystogram should be performed to exclude a bladder injury. If a catheter cannot be passed, then a delayed CT cystogram is the only option. Urethral injuries are usually confirmed by ascending urethrography, which is often performed by the trauma team.

Interventional aspects

The only radiological treatment option to consider is vascular intervention in the haemodynamically unstable patient. It is therefore absolutely imperative that this should be considered when reporting any pelvic injury and always maintaining a low threshold for seeking help from the interventionalists.

Acute reporting

- Is there evidence of active bleeding? Does the pattern fit with anterior compression/vertical shear injuries, which are often haemodynamically unstable, or a lateral compression injury which is usually stable?

Extremity trauma

Summary

Protocol: Non-contrast examination with thin (1 mm) slice thickness and two plane reformats.

What to look for: Correlate with plain film.

Report: Confirm the presence of a fracture, describe its true extent.

Extremity fractures classically are assessed by plain radiographs. With the advent of multidetector CT (MDCT) with good quality reformats, CT is now routinely used to fully characterize virtually any complex fracture. CT primarily looks at the articular surfaces, the degree of fragmentation and the possibility of reconstruction. The presence of intra-articular fragments should be noted to ensure that these are removed expeditiously.

Protocol and technique

Contrast enhancement: Non-contrast examination with thin (1 mm) slice thickness and two plane reformats.

What to look for on CT

- It is essential with any extremity injury to look at the plain radiographs to gain an initial overview. The CT dataset will allow reformatted images in any required plane (Figs 3.9, 3.10). As with plain radiographs, at least two planes are often necessary to fully appreciate the injury with a third or even a curved plane sometimes necessary.

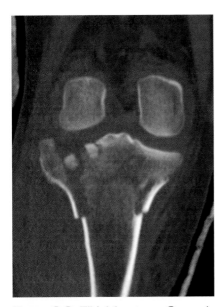

Figure 3.9: Tibial fracture. Coronal image showing a tibial fracture. The extent and degree of fragmentation is clearly demonstrated.

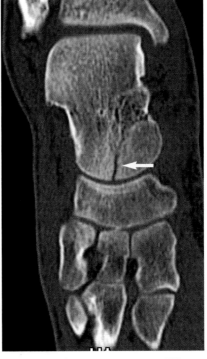

Figure 3.10: Talus fracture. CT shows the sagittal split (arrow) and confirmed that there were no other fractures present.

- The shoulder, hip and elbow can be difficult to assess and for injuries to those structures, a quick 3D reformat is often helpful to fully orientate yourself before carrying out the detailed report.
- The other situation where CT has gained wide acceptance is when there is the suspicion of a fracture on the plain radiograph but the surgeon requires definitive proof to guide further management. If a fracture is confirmed, its full extent can be documented.

Acute reporting

- Clinicians require a description of the extent of the injury and any articular surface involvement.
- Where there is doubt about a fracture, confirmation of its presence is the priority. The converse also applies when a fracture proves to be far more extensive than initially appreciated.
- There are countless classification systems for fractures, but rather than learn them all, it is advisable to discuss with your local orthopaedic surgeons which ones they find of practical value.

Recommended reading

Canadian c-spine rule. *JAMA* 2001;**286**:1841–8.

Canadian c-spine rule validated. *N Engl J Med* 2003;**349**:2510–18.

Denis F. The 3 column spine and its significance in the classification of acute thoraco-lumbar spinal injuries. *Spine* 1983;**8**:817.

Harris JH, Mirvis SE. *The Radiology of the Acute Spine*, 3rd edn. Philadelphia: Lippincott Williams and Wilkins, 1996.

Judet R, Judet J, Letournel E. Fractures of the acetabulum: classification and surgical approaches for open reduction. *J Bone Joint Surg (Am)* 1964; **46**:1615–46.

Nuñez DB Jr, Ahmad AA, Coin CG, et al. Clearing the cervical spine in multiple trauma victims: a time-effective protocol using helical CT. *Emerg Radiol* 1994;273–8.

Obenauer S, Alamo L, Herold T, et al. Imaging skeletal anatomy of injured cervical spine specimens: comparison of single-slice vs. multi-slice helical CT. *Eur Radiol* 2002;**12**:2107–11.

Blunt aortic trauma

Summary

Protocol: IV contrast, triphasic scan, ECG gating.

What to look for: Periaortic haemorrhage, aortic pseudoaneurysm, intimal luminal flap, contrast extravasation, abnormal aortic contour.

Report: Site, vessel diameter, degree of injury/vessel disruption.

Blunt aortic trauma is most commonly seen in the setting of a high veloc-ity motor vehicle accident. Fifteen per cent of patients with injury to the aorta or great vessels survive the initial incident and make it to hospital. Of these, 50% die within 24 hours. Without prompt diagnosis and treat-ment, 90% will die within 4 months. With appropriate diagnosis and treatment, 80% will survive

Protocol and technique

Contrast enhancement: Non-contrast (5 mm), arterial phase (1–1.25 mm) and portal venous phase (2.5–5 mm) scans should be per-formed with coverage from lung apices to diaphragms. 100 ml of IV con-trast ideally delivered at 5 ml/s. ECG-gated scanning should always be used if available. This minimizes movement artefact at the aortic root.

With modern polytrauma imaging, dedicated aortic protocols are infre-quently used as part of the initial imaging of the trauma patient when, more typically, a compromise best-fit coverage of the head, spine, chest abdomen and pelvis is performed. Chest coverage is usually done during the arterial phase with abdominal imaging favouring the portal venous phase. Protocols can be modified depending on the mechanism of injury or any specific clinical concerns.

What to look for on CT

- *Periaortic mediastinal haemorrhage:* This is usually seen at the level of the aortic arch and proximal descending aorta. Occasionally, haemorrhage tracks down below the diaphragm. In the trauma situa-tion, haematoma isolated to the anterior or posterior mediastinum and not in direct contact with the aorta is seldom associated with major arterial injury. In rare cases, periaortic haemorrhage may be absent despite significant aortic injury.
- *Aortic pseudoaneurysm:* Look for a rounded bulge from the aortic lumen that typically displays irregular margins. A pseudoaneurysm usually arises from the anterior aspect of the proximal descending aorta at the level of the left main bronchus. A linear intimal flap typi-cally projects across the base. When reporting a pseudoaneurysm, not-ing the relationship of the point of origin of the pseudoaneurysm and closest branch vessel is crucial to planning surgical intervention.
- *Aortic contour and calibre variation:* A sudden change in aortic calibre or irregular aortic shape should alert you to the possibility of a circumferential tear or a dissection.
- *Intimal luminal flap/thrombus:* Look for a thin low attenuation intimal flap projecting into the lumen. It is crucial to use wide viewing windows to give yourself any chance of seeing the flap. Mural throm-

bus often forms in association with the flap along the aortic wall and this may form a source of embolus.

- **Contrast extravasation:** This is rarely seen on CT but when present, death is imminent from exsanguination. Extensive mediastinal haematoma, bulging of mediastinal pleura, and displacement of trachea and oesophagus may also be present.
- **Mass effect:** Mass effect is a more important sign when interpreting the chest radiograph, but displacement of oesophagus, trachea and nasogastric tube to the right should all be documented.
- **Mimics/pitfalls:** There are a few mimics of blunt aortic injury:
  - ☐ A ductus diverticulum results in a focal convex bulge along the anteroinferior surface of the isthmic region of the aortic arch.
  - ☐ An aortic spindle can be seen as a mild fusiform enlargement between the left subclavian artery and the attachment of the ductus arteriosus.
  - ☐ A ductus remnant results in a small irregularity in the aortic wall and is usually calcified.
- **Other pitfalls:**
  - ☐ Aortic injury can occur without mediastinal haematoma or haemorrhage and usually results from cervicothoracic spinal injury or sternal fracture. Bleeding is confined to the posterior or anterior mediastinum, respectively.
  - ☐ An atypical location of injury is seen in 10% of patients. Review areas should include the peridiaphragmatic aorta, the aortic arch and the ascending aorta. Look for signs of other mediastinal injury such as oesophageal tear/rupture.
  - ☐ Do not mistake areas of atelectatic lung located adjacent to the dorsal aorta as contrast extravasation. If in doubt, rescan the area to see if extravasated contrast has increased in volume; if atelectasis, there will have been rapid contrast wash out. You may identify an air bronchogram within a segment of ateletasis.

Acute reporting

- It is vital to record the number, location and extent of injuries.
- Record the diameter of the aorta/great vessels above and below the site of injury, as well as the length of injury along the major vascular axis. This allows planning for both open or endovascular repair.
- The type of pathology and any anatomical variants should be recorded.

Recommended reading

Fishman EK, Horton KM, Johnson PT. Multidetector CT and three-dimensional CT angiography for suspected vascular trauma of the extremities. *Radiographics* 2008;**28**:653–65; discussion 665–6.

Adult abdominal trauma

Summary

Protocol: Oral contrast is not a requirement for blunt polytrauma imaging. For penetrating trauma, oral and rectal contrast is advisable. IV contrast with imaging in portal venous phase. CT cystogram when major pelvic trauma demonstrated.

What to look for: Free fluid/haemoperitoneum, free gas; injury to solid organs, bowel and bone; active haemorrhage.

Report: Location and severity of injuries. Need for intervention.

MDCT is the primary imaging choice for the acute evaluation of abdominal injury. Other techniques such as focused ultrasound may have a role in some circumstances, but CT provides the most comprehensive whole body coverage in the shortest time scale for most trauma situations. Abdominal trauma imaging is now less commonly performed in isolation but typically is just one part of a global polytrauma study that will include the head, spine, chest, abdomen and pelvis.

Abdominal injury generally results from one of two mechanisms, either penetrating or blunt trauma. Fractured bones, gun-shot and knife injuries are the commoner causes of penetrating trauma. Blunt trauma may result from deceleration or concussion events. Deceleration leads to differential movement of fixed and non-fixed structures that may lead to solid organ injury. An example of this type of injury is the liver laceration located along the attachment of the ligamentum teres. Compression or concussion injuries result from either a direct blow to the body, or structures being crushed against a fixed object, e.g. lap belt injuries. The transient increase in intra-abdominal pressure caused by these forces can result in organ rupture.

The role of CT in the 'unstable' trauma patient has been a source of much debate and disagreement over the years. Patients are often unstable because they are actively bleeding. Acute haemorrhage is rapidly detected by MDCT and can be promptly treated by interventional radiologists, thereby avoiding unnecessary surgery. Faster scanners producing whole body coverage within a very short period of time largely negate the old fashioned 'doughnut of death' philosophy. Conventional triage plain films can also be replaced by the rapid whole body CT package. When emergency surgical intervention is required, a detailed radiological review can be ongoing at the diagnostic workstation or PACS monitor as the patient is transferred to theatre. A preoperative indication of the location, severity and extent of injury can be invaluable for surgical planning and decision making.

Protocol and technique

Contrast enhancement:

- **Oral contrast:** Most trauma centres have moved away from the routine use of oral contrast in blunt trauma imaging. It is important to ensure that the trauma patient's stay in the CT unit is as short as possible, and modern CT technology with thin-section reconstruction and multiplanar reformatted imaging has reduced the need for oral contrast with its inherent delays, irrespective of the means of delivery. However, for penetrating injury to the abdomen, oral contrast is useful for detecting perforation of stomach or small bowel.
- **Rectal contrast:** The use of rectal/colonic contrast improves the detection of large bowel injury in penetrating trauma, and most trauma centres would advocate its routine use when such an injury is being assessed. A litre of 2–3% contrast is delivered by gravity feed via a rectal catheter.
- **IV contrast:** Mandatory unless specifically contraindicated. 100–150 ml of contrast with standard image acquisition during the portal venous phase of contrast enhancement.

Variations to standard post contrast protocol:

1. When active bleeding is suspected on clinical grounds (appropriate history/mechanism/poor haemodynamics), a non-contrast and arterial phase series can be added to the protocol.
2. When haemorrhage is detected on the portal venous phase acquisition or solid organ injury is identified, an immediate repeat series is recommended to show contrast accumulation and help differentiate between active bleeding and traumatic arteriovenous communication. In the former situation, the volume and density of the extravasated contrast will increase, whereas with the latter, contrast wash out mirroring adjacent intact vascular structures will be apparent.
3. With renal injury, a delayed series at about 5–10 min is recommended to identify extravasation of opacified urine from damaged calyces, renal pelvis or ureter.
4. **CT cystogram:** Pelvic fractures are associated with a high incidence of bladder injury and a CT cystogram should be added to the protocol if bladder injury is suspected. This technique has a very high sensitivity and specificity for the detection of bladder injury. Obtaining delayed images after opacified urine fills the bladder is a poorer alternative option.

Slice collimation: 2.5 mm axial reconstructions for general abdominal images, with selected thinner section reconstruction for the evaluation of spinal structures and multiplanar reformatted images.

What to look for on CT

General rules for trauma image review:

1. It is imperative to carefully review all images with a variety of windows and imaging planes using a dedicated workstation. Soft tissue, lung and bone settings are standard requirements. The workstation 'invert' function or the use of 'wide' rather than lung windows improves the detection of free gas.
2. A systematic approach is necessary to ensure all anatomy and organ systems are covered during the image review. Polytrauma image review is typically accompanied by multiple clinical firms imposing their own specific demands on the reporting radiologist. Unless a disciplined systematic approach is followed, the potential to miss significant injury is high. We find the use of a dedicated trauma reporting proforma a useful aid to ensure all areas of potential injury are evaluated, as well as providing an easily understood summary of the key findings.
3. Abdominal injuries generally follow predictable patterns and relate to 'corridors of impact'. Image review should therefore pay particular attention to adjacent anatomy when an injury is detected. For example, a splenic injury should lead to careful review of the left kidney, tail of pancreas, left chest wall and diaphragm.
4. The concept of 'satisfaction of search' is especially important with trauma imaging. The finding of one injury needs the careful exclusion of other abnormalities (Fig. 3.11).

Specific abdominal organ injury

Spleen

The spleen is the most frequently injured solid organ and CT has an accuracy of up to 98% for the detection of splenic injuries, which include a shattered spleen (multiple crossing lacerations), disruption of splenic hilar vessels, parenchymal lacerations, capsular tears and contusions.

What to look for on CT

- *Splenic haematoma:* Subcapsular haematomas appear as crescentic low attenuation areas along the margins of the spleen that may flatten or indent the splenic contour. Parenchymal haematomas may be isodense or even hypodense (compared to spleen) if imaged in the early post-traumatic period. Splenic haematomas are unique because of the spleen's potential to bleed and rebleed, leading to the characteristic layered or onion skin appearance on CT.

- **Splenic laceration:** These appear as linear low attenuation parenchymal defects and are almost always associated with haemoperitoneum. A laceration becomes a 'fracture' when it traverses two capsular surfaces. Normal anatomical splenic clefts can mimic lacerations. Look for a 'sentinel clot' that may indicate a parenchymal injury not immediately visible and will help differentiate between true lacerations and anatomical clefts. Sentinel clots generally have attenuation values over 60 HU when compared with the typically lower density haemoperitoneum.
- **Active splenic haemorrhage:** The demonstration of contrast extravasation indicates active haemorrhage and a second acquisition should be performed to differentiate between a traumatic pseudoaneurysm and active bleeding.
- **Delayed splenic rupture:** Delayed rupture is almost unique to splenic injury. Typically this presents more than 48 hours after the initial injury and is reported in up to 20% of all blunt trauma cases.

Liver

Liver trauma can be associated with high morbidity and mortality. Advances in CT technology and interventional radiology techniques have contributed to a major shift in focus from surgical to non-surgical management.

What to look for on CT (Fig. 3.12)

- **Haemoperitoneum:** A common finding with most solid organ injuries. Injuries involving segment VII and the bare area of liver may be associated with retroperitoneal rather than intraperitoneal haemorrhage.
- **Lacerations:** These appear as irregular linear or branching low attenuation defects which tend to follow anatomical planes. Deep lacerations (>3 cm) located around the porta hepatis have an increased association with biliary complications. Lacerations that extend up to, or closely approximate, hepatic vessels must be considered high risk for causing vascular injury. Be careful not to confuse normal liver clefts with lacerations. These are often found along the medial aspect of segments 5 and 6.

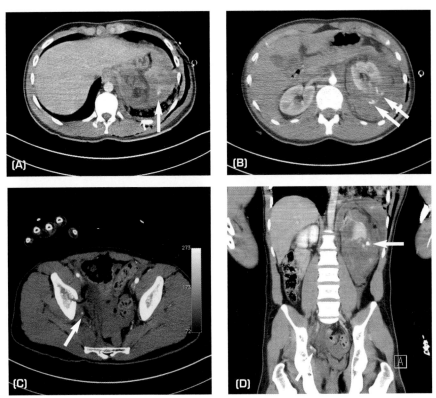

Figure 3.11: Multifocal injuries following a road traffic accident. (A)
Hypoperfused spleen, perhaps reflecting splenic pedicle injury. Active splenic
parenchymal bleeding indicated by the focus of high attenuation (arrow) that
shows comparable density to the aorta. **(B)** Left kidney laceration with
further active contrast extravasation (arrows) and extensive perirenal
haematoma. **(C)** Pelvic haematoma and a further bleeding point adjacent to
the iliac fracture (arrow). **(D)** Coronal image confirming location of the renal
and pelvic bleeding points (arrows). Compare the density of splenic
enhancement with that of liver.

■ ***Subcapsular and parenchymal haematoma:*** Haematomas
appear as areas of increased density (40–60 HU), the actual density
depending on the age of the clot and whether bleeding is ongoing or
rebleeding has occurred. A subcapsular haematoma is recognized as
an elliptical collection located between the liver capsule and the adjacent enhancing liver that exerts mass effect on the underlying liver
margin. This contrasts with a simple haemoperitoneum or uncomplicated ascites that do not alter the contour of adjacent structures.
Intrahepatic haematomas show no significant enhancement unless

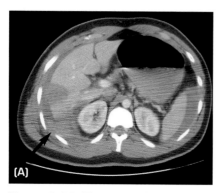 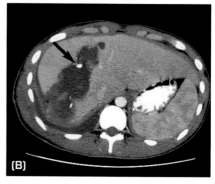

Figure 3.12: Traumatic hepatic laceration and haemoperitoneum.
(A) Low attenuation wedge-shaped defect reflecting laceration and haematoma in right lobe following blunt trauma. Note associated high-density haemoperitoneum (arrow). **(B)** Gun-shot injury with bullet path traversing right and left lobes. Arrow indicates a bullet fragment. Patchy splenic enhancement pattern reflects the arterial phase of this image and is a normal finding not indicative of splenic injury.

active bleeding is present and a second image acquisition would confirm contrast accumulation in this circumstance. As with all solid organ injuries, look for the 'sentinel clot sign'. The densest haematoma usually lies adjacent to the site of injury.

- **Active haemorrhage:** Acute haemorrhage may be life-threatening and hence its detection is vital as potential treatment by embolization can avoid the need for open surgery. Look for contrast extravasation with delayed imaging showing contrast accumulation rather than contrast wash out with time. Active extravasation can be differentiated from clotted blood by assessing its CT density. Contrast has typical density values of between 90 and 200 HU, whereas clotted blood densities range between 30 and 80 HU (Fig. 3.13).

- **Hepatic venous injury:** Venous injuries can be life-threatening and may require prompt surgical treatment. Venous injury should be suspected when hepatic lacerations or haematomas extend towards major hepatic veins or the inferior vena cava (IVC). For practical purposes, a laceration extending in close proximity to a major vessel should be assumed to involve the vessel.

- **Periportal oedema:** Look for linear low attenuation densities paralleling the portal vein and its branches. These are typically seen following fluid resuscitation of a shocked patient. Occasionally, dissecting periportal haemorrhage can have similar appearances.

- **Complications of liver injury:** These are generally recognized on follow-up imaging rather than during the initial diagnostic study, and

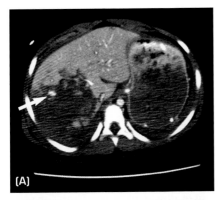

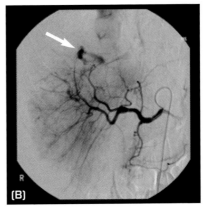

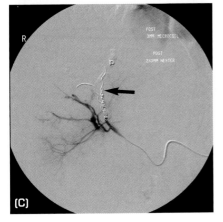

Figure 3.13: Liver injury with active bleeding. (A) Axial section shows focal high attenuation contrast extravasation within a major injury to the right liver. (B) Subsequent angiography shows continuing active bleeding (arrow), (C) successfully treated with coil embolization (arrow). (Angiography images courtesy of Dr Simon McPherson, Consultant Vascular Radiologist, Leeds Teaching Hospitals, Leeds, UK.)

include abscess, pseudoaneurysm formation, and biliary complications such as haemobilia, biloma and biliary peritonitis. Bile leakage leads to biloma formation and potential liver necrosis. Look for an enlarging well-circumscribed, low attenuation collection after liver trauma. Most traumatic bilomas regress spontaneously, but drainage may be required if there is accompanying or worsening pain, obstructive symptoms or signs of infection.

Renal tract

Renal tract injuries are found in up to 10% of patients with significant abdominal trauma but up to 95% of these can be managed conservatively. The spectrum of injury includes contusion, subcapsular haematoma, laceration, shattered kidney and renal artery avulsion or occlusion. Look for location of injury, type (contusion, laceration), severity, perirenal haemorrhage and presence of urinary extravasation.

What to look for on CT (Fig. 3.14)

- ***Contusion and haematoma:*** Renal parenchymal contusions present as foci of reduced parenchymal enhancement while subcapsular haematomas vary in attenuation depending on their age. When the renal capsule is disrupted, blood enters the perinephric space.

- ***Laceration:*** Renal lacerations appear as linear, low attenuation defects in the parenchyma and may be superficial (<1 cm) or deep (>1 cm). Deep lacerations involving the pelvicalyceal system can result in urine extravasation and urinoma formation.

- ***Active haemorrhage:*** Active haemorrhage is diagnosed by identifying focal contrast enhancement associated with a laceration or haematoma. Management is generally endovascular and therefore the interventional radiologist should be alerted at the earliest opportunity. Haemorrhage tends to track into surrounding tissues and has a linear or infiltrative appearance, contrasting with a pseudoaneurysm which tends to be more focal and rounded. Renal arterial avulsion typically results in minimal haematoma due to intense vascular spasm limiting the blood loss. Significant haematoma is more typically found with renal venous laceration, reflecting the vein's inability to contract in response to injury.

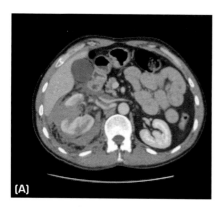 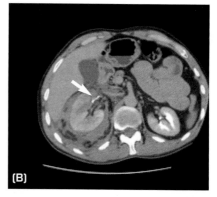

(A)   (B)

Figure 3.14: Traumatic renal injury. (A) Contrast enhanced image shows fracture of mid pole of right kidney. Note intra- and peri-renal haematoma. (B) A 5 minute delayed image revealed no urinary contrast extravastion but showing lymphatic contrast excretion (arrow).

- **_Renal infarction:_** Occurs secondary to thrombosis or laceration of a segmental renal arterial branch: Infarcts typically appear as non-enhancing peripheral wedge-shaped parenchymal defects.
- **_Urinary extravasation:_** Detection requires delayed imaging 5–10 minutes after intravenous contrast administration. Urinary extravasation resolves spontaneously in a high percentage (up to 87%) of patients. Follow-up CT will be indicated in patients who develop signs of sepsis with CT-guided aspiration or drainage of urinomas often required.

Urinary bladder

Bladder injuries occur in 8% of all patients with pelvic fractures. While intraperitoneal ruptures (20% of cases) require surgical repair, the more common extraperitoneal ruptures may be treated conservatively. Mixed intraperitoneal and extraperitoneal patterns can be present, and CT cystography is the recommended imaging technique when bladder injury is suspected or likely. With intraperitoneal rupture, look for contrast accumulation in the lower peritoneal reflections, outlining pelvic small bowel loops and extending up the paracolic gutters (Figs 3.15, 3.16).

Pancreas

Pancreatic trauma is one of the less common abdominal injuries but is associated with a mortality rate of up to 20%. Early diagnosis is crucial,

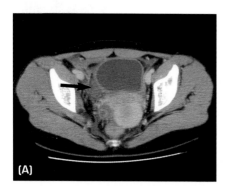 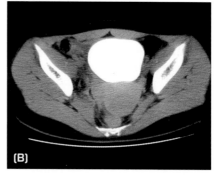

Figure 3.15: CT cystogram. (A) Part of trauma series indicates fluid around urinary bladder (arrow), raising concerns of bladder wall injury. **(B)** The subsequent CT cystogram confirms no contrast leak from the bladder, giving a high degree of certainty that no significant bladder wall injury is present.

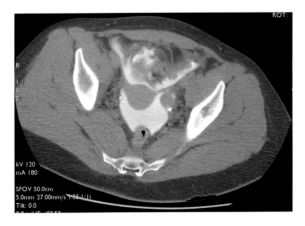

Figure 3.16: Traumatic bladder rupture. CT cystography showing intraperitoneal rupture as well as intraluminal haematoma.

as delayed complications, such as pancreatitis, pseudocyst formation, sepsis and haemorrhage, may be devastating and largely account for the high morbidity and mortality. Most major complications result from disruption of the pancreatic duct. Since the pancreas is rarely injured in isolation, careful review of adjacent anatomical structures is essential.

- The spectrum of pancreatic injuries consists of contusion, fracture and duct disruption. Carefully review the anterior pancreatic margin looking for irregularity or disruption to the normal curved contour. Focal enlargement, peripancreatic fat stranding or peripancreatic fluid are other key signs. Peripancreatic fluid is typically of low attenuation and tends to contrast with any adjacent higher density haemoperitoneum (Fig. 3.17).
- If a trauma patient develops unexplained delayed epigastric or back pain, fever or hyperamylasaemia, repeat imaging using a dedicated pancreatic protocol may reveal a pancreatic injury that may not have been apparent or not appreciated on the initial study.

Bowel and mesentery

Bowel and mesenteric injuries are found at laparotomy in 5% of blunt abdominal trauma. The commonest injured segments of bowel are the **jejunum** and **ileum**, followed by the colon and duodenum, and occasionally the stomach. The prompt detection and treatment of bowel and mesenteric injuries is critical as associated peritonitis and ongoing haemorrhage result in increased morbidity and mortality.

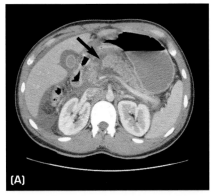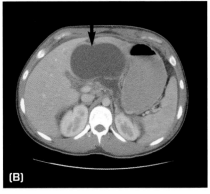

(A) **(B)**

Figure 3.17: Transected pancreas. (A) Fracture through the pancreatic neck (arrow) with adjacent peripancreatic fluid and ascites in a patient who experienced blunt trauma to the abdomen. **(B)** A well-demarcated fluid collection anterior to the pancreas (arrow) in a different patient, again following blunt trauma. This image was part of a follow-up examination. Note the typical simple fluid density of pancreatic juice which often shows significant density differences to the more generalized haemoperitoneum found in patients with multiple intra-abdominal injuries.

What to look for on CT

- **Contusion:** Areas of focal or asymmetrical mural thickening indicating mural haematoma. More generalized bowel wall thickening is a non-specific sign in the trauma setting, particularly in the shocked patient, but focal bowel wall thickening is more worrisome (Fig. 3.18).
- **Perforation and transection:** Perforation should be considered when extraluminal gas, extraluminal bowel content including faeces, or extravasated oral contrast is detected. Unexplained intraperitoneal fluid should always trigger a careful search for bowel injury. Wide windows or use of the invert function will aid the detection of free gas. Early signs can be very subtle and tiny foci of gas or small mesenteric triangles of unexplained fluid may be the only findings (Fig. 3.19).
- Look for associated soft tissue abnormalities, such as haematoma formation in the subcutaneous fat or focal abdominal wall muscle enlargement, that will indicate the site of impact and therefore point to areas of related mesenteric or bowel injury.
- When the initial CT shows only non-specific signs, and bowel injury remains a strong clinical possibility, follow-up imaging should be performed in 6–8 hours, assuming the patient does not require immediate surgery.

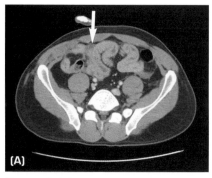

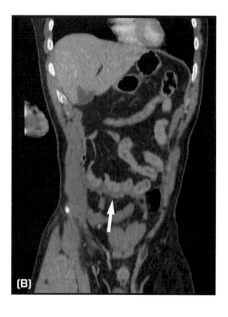

Figure 3.18: Small bowel injury. Motorcyclist presenting with peritonitic abdomen and fractured femur following collision with a car. **(A)** Axial and **(B)** coronal sections showing abnormal small bowel loops with high-density mural thickening and perienteric fluid extending into the adjacent mesentery (arrows). Note poor small bowel wall mural clarity due to adjacent perienteric fluid on coronal section. At operation, extensive devascularization of the small bowel mesentery and multiple shearing injuries to large and small bowel were found.

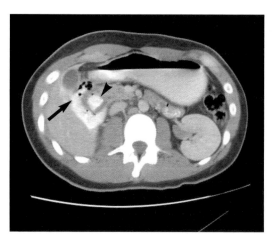

Figure 3.19: Duodenal trauma. A 17-year-old male presented with abdominal pain following blunt abdominal injury. Extraluminal gas and contrast extravasation (arrow) indicates duodenal injury. Arrowhead identifies contrast within duodenal lumen. An example of the benefits of selective use of oral contrast in abdominal trauma.

- Signs of mesenteric vascular injuries include:
  - ☐ **Active contrast extravasation** from mesenteric vessels.
  - ☐ Abnormal vessel morphology such as **vascular beading**.
  - ☐ **Abrupt termination** of a mesenteric vessel.

- ☐ Secondary effects such as **bowel infarct** may be found but early detection can be difficult on CT.
  - ☐ Less severe mesenteric injury can result in more subtle localized increased mesenteric fat density, a finding which may be more readily appreciated on coronal reformatted images.
- Major disruption to the greater omentum and lesser sac may occur with crush injuries to the epigastrium. Look for pockets of fluid, haematoma and active bleeding in a distribution that may not conform to expected pathways of fluid spread. Carefully review those sections of bowel which lie within the corridor of crush injury, such as the transverse colon and stomach.

Gallbladder

The gallbladder is the most commonly injured component of the biliary tract with a reported incidence of 2–3% in blunt trauma. Injury rarely occurs in isolation and is usually associated with liver (90%), splenic (50%) and duodenal (50%) trauma and because of this, gallbladder injuries are often overlooked or not considered. The commoner forms of injury include contusions and haematoma, either intra-luminal mural or both.

What to look for on CT

- Look for focal thickening or reduced definition of the gallbladder wall. A collapsed gallbladder may indicate perforation or avulsion, particularly if associated with a pericholecystic collection.
- Avulsion of the gallbladder pedicle may result in major blood loss due to laceration of the cystic artery, so an unexplained haematoma adjacent to the gallbladder fossa should raise concerns.
- When the gallbladder lies in an atypical location, this should raise concern of gallbladder pedicular damage.

Shock (Figs 3.20–3.22)

The CT findings will reflect the severity of shock but look for a collapsed inferior vena cava, hyperenhancing adrenal glands and generalized increased enhancement along with mural thickening of the small bowel. With increasing severity of shock, organ hypoperfusion will develop. The kidneys, spleen and liver are particularly vulnerable to hypoperfusion insult and patchy abnormal enhancement patterns will ensue as the blood supply to these structures begins to shut down. Capsular vessel supply may be maintained until late, leading to rim enhancement of otherwise hypoperfused organs.

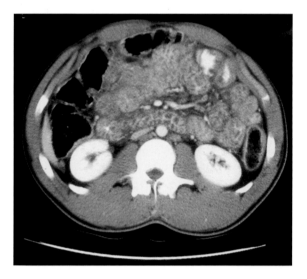

Figure 3.20: Shock bowel. Note global mural thickening of all small bowel loops shown on this section.

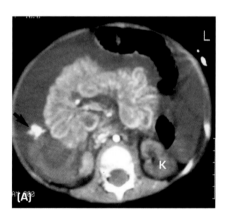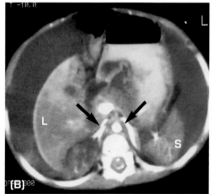

Figure 3.21: Severe shock. Many of the CT findings in severe shock are illustrated in this example of a severely injured child who should never have reached a CT scanner. Note hyperenhancing small bowel mural thickening in **(A)** with arrow indicating active contrast extravasation from a mesenteric injury. Hyperenhancing adrenal glands (**B**, arrows) along with hypoperfusion of spleen (S), kidneys and liver (L) indicate the severity of the patient's compromised circulation.

Acute reporting of abdominal trauma CT

- Be structured and systematic in your approach, listing all injuries and commenting on severity and extent.

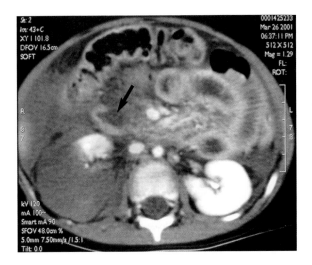

Figure 3.22: Shock. Child with traumatic duodenal rupture (arrow). Note haemoperitoneum, hyperenhancing thickened bowel wall and right renal injury.

- Try and give yourself sufficient time to carefully review the study before coming to your final conclusion. However, the time available for image review will be largely determined by the patient's clinical status.
- Some emergency clinicians prefer the radiologist to also comment on anatomical structures or areas that have been cleared of injury, in addition to itemizing structures that are injured.
- Identify active bleeding and inform the surgeons and interventional radiologist at the earliest opportunity.
- Indicate areas of uncertainty and discuss the role of early repeat or planned follow-up imaging.
- Seek specialist radiological opinion if injuries outside your experience are shown and management depends on a specific diagnosis.

Recommended reading

Harris AC, Zwirewich CV, Lyburn ID, Torreggiani WC, Marchinkow LO. CT finding in blunt renal trauma. *Radiographics* 2001;**21** (Suppl):S201–14.

Kumar MM, Venkataramannapa M, Venkataratnam I, Kumar NV, Babji K Prospective evaluation of blunt abdominal trauma by computed tomography. *Indian J Radiol Imaging* 2005;**15**:167–73 from: http://www.ijri.org/text.asp?2005/15/2/167/28794.

Lubner M, Menias C, Rucker C, et al. Blood in the belly: CT findings of hemoperitoneum. *Radiographics* 2007;**27**:109–25.

Patel SV, Spencer JA, El-hasani S, Sheridan MB. Imaging of pancreatic trauma. *Br J Radiol* 1998;**71**:985–990.

Shanmuganathan K, Mirvis SE, Chiu WC, Kileen KL, Dutton RP. Triple-contrast helical CT in penetrating torso trauma: a prospective study to determine peritoneal violation and the need for laparotomy. *AJR Am J Roentgenol* 2001;**177**:1247–56.

Yoon W, Jeong YY, Kim JK, et al. CT in blunt liver trauma. *Radiographics* 2005;**25**:87–104.

Trauma in children

Although the CT appearances of the common childhood injuries have many similarities to those found in adults, it is imperative that radiologists recognize those anatomical features unique to children, as well as appreciating the pathophysiological processes that affect children who are victims of trauma. In children, a force directed towards a given body area will often result in a more significant injury when compared to an adult.

- Children have a greater body surface area relative to their weight. The distribution of injury will be more extensive, leading to a greater incidence of multifocal trauma.
- A relatively greater surface area results in children experiencing greater heat loss compared to adults, a factor that needs to be addressed while the patient is on the CT table.
- The paediatric thorax is a compliant structure and the predominantly cartilaginous rib cage affords protection. This compressibility has the advantage of dissipating the force of impact but at the same time can be problematic because it reduces the likelihood of an external injury despite the presence of significant internal pathology.
- The paediatric mediastinum is a more mobile structure than the adult equivalent, which increases the likelihood of significant ventilatory or circulatory collapse in the presence of a tension pneumothorax.
- Isolated chest injury is relatively uncommon, but its presence increases the likelihood of multisystem trauma by 10-fold.
- Children have less well-developed abdominal musculature and less subcutaneous fat than adults, both of which lead to reduced protection of intra-abdominal contents and an increased vulnerability to injury.
- The more anteriorly located liver and spleen are at increased risk from forces directed at the upper abdomen.
- The kidneys are more mobile and less protected by the lower posterior ribs, leaving them vulnerable to deceleration injury.

Paediatric cervical spine injury

Sixty to 80% of vertebral injuries in children occur in the cervical spine and of these, 70% occur above the C3 level. Thirty to 40% of injuries in this age group include spinal cord injury without radiographic abnormality (SCIWORA). Therefore, the absence of a radiographic abnormality in a symptomatic child should *not* falsely reassure the clinician as injury to the non-osseous elements of the paediatric spine can result in significant instability. When suspected, MRI is the tool of choice to evaluate both spinal cord integrity and soft tissue injury.

Certain clinical criteria should prompt a request for imaging: midline cervical tenderness, altered level of alertness, evidence of intoxication, neurological abnormality and painful distracting injury. Remember that in children under age 2 years, some of these criteria are difficult to establish.

Protocol and technique

Contrast: Not required.

Slice collimation: Thin slices (1 mm).

What to look for on CT

- A child's cervical spine has some unique anatomical characteristics that the radiologist must be aware of when interpreting the CT images:
  - ☐ The spine will be incompletely ossified.
  - ☐ The facet joints are flatter and more horizontally orientated.
  - ☐ The basilar odontoid synchondrosis fuses at 3–7 years.
  - ☐ The apical odontoid epiphysis fuses at 5–7 years.
  - ☐ The posterior arch of C1 fuses at age 4 years.
  - ☐ The anterior arch fuses at age 7–10 years.
  - ☐ The preodontoid space may normally measure up to 4–5 mm before age 10 years.
  - ☐ The size of the prevertebral space may vary with respiration.
- *Atlantoaxial injury:*
  - ☐ Is 10 times more common in children under 10 years.
  - ☐ Abnormal alignment of the occiput, C1 and/or C2 is best appreciated on coronal views.
  - ☐ Atlanto-occipital dissociation is two to three times more common in children and is often fatal at the time of injury. Concomitant anterior translation of the occiput on C1 causes an increase in the BC/OA ratio (ratio of the distance between the basion and the posterior arch of C1 divided by the distance between the opisthion and the anterior arch of C1; normal ratio <1).
- *Fractures:* Certain fractures may be more or less common in children:
  - ☐ An **odontoid fracture** is much less common in younger children when compared to adolescents and adults.
  - ☐ The **os odontoideum** results from a fracture through the odontoid synchodrosis prior to its normal fusion at age 5–6 years. It is more often present in children with skeletal dysplasias, and may be a source of instability.
  - ☐ **Ossiculum terminale**, a result of non-fusion of the distal ossification center, is not clinically significant.

Differential diagnosis

- Certain normal variants may mimic injury, and knowledge of these entities is imperative for accurate radiographic assessment of the paediatric cervical spine.
- The epiphyses of the spinous process tips may mimic fractures.

Pseudosubluxation of C2 on C3 may be present in up to 40% of patients under age 18 years (PIX). The **spinolaminar (Swischuk's) line** can be used to differentiate true subluxation from pseudosubluxation. This line should parallel the anterior cortical margin of the spinous process of C1 down through that of C3. If, at C2, this line crosses the anterior cortical margin of the C2 spinous process or it is off by less than 2 mm, and no fracture is present, the patient has pseudosubluxation.

Certain pre-existing pathologies such as juvenile rheumatoid arthritis, acquired anomalies such as old mature fractures, or congenital anomalies such as Down's syndrome, may have challenging anatomy that increases the difficulty of the clinical and radiological assessment. Ten to 20% of Down's syndrome patients have excessive laxity of the transverse ligament, a finding also common in patients with Morquio, Ehlers-Danlos and Marfan syndrome. Grisel syndrome describes instability secondary to adjacent soft tissue inflammation.

Non-accidental paediatric trauma

It is the responsibility of the radiologist to recognize injury patterns that point to a non-accidental aetiology. Overcalling non-accidental injury can put unnecessary emotional and social stress on the patient and family, while undercalling risks placing a child back into an unsafe environment.

Multiple injuries, particularly when of different ages, should always suggest a diagnosis of non-accidental injury. When severe injury is found, the history obtained from the patient and carer must adequately explain the degree of force required to produce such an injury. Common false histories include a child rolling off a couch, a sibling stepping on the child, or a carer rolling onto a child in bed. These mechanisms may not adequately account for the force needed to inflict significant intracranial pathology. Finally, whenever the CT findings suggest possible physical abuse in a child younger than age 2 years of age, the radiologist must ensure that a skeletal survey is performed. For children older than 5 years, the survey is of limited value. Children between ages 2 and 5 years must be handled on a case-by-case basis.

Central nervous system injury

Central nervous system (CNS) injury is the leading cause of death from abusive injury in children. CNS injuries may result from direct impact, violent shaking, or a combination of these. Infants younger than 6 months are at the highest risk for shaking injury, and certain anatomical features in children predispose them to acceleration/deceleration injury. Children are small, light weight and easy to shake. The head is proportionally large relative to the body and they have poor neck control.

What to look for on CT

- **Subdural haemorrhage:**
  - ☐ Is the most common consequence of shaking.
  - ☐ Cerebrospinal fluid (CSF) dilution, haematocrit level and coagulation status affect the CT appearance, and the typical findings used to age a haematoma in an adult do *not* apply in children.
  - ☐ Injuries of the same age may look different; therefore, dating intracranial haemorrhage accurately is not possible unless comparison imaging is available.
- **Subdural hygroma:**
  - ☐ May develop after 12–24 h.
  - ☐ Is of CSF density due to leakage of CSF from the subarachnoid space.
- **Ischaemic injury:**
  - ☐ Shaking injuries show a high correlation with damage to the parenchyma.
  - ☐ Loss of grey–white matter differentiation or a relative decrease in density of the cerebrum when compared to the cerebellum may be seen in acute injuries.
  - ☐ Ischaemic patterns that do not correspond to a vascular territory should raise concern.
  - ☐ Simultaneous subarachnoid haemorrhage is present in over 50% of cases.
- **Fractures:**
  - ☐ CT is sensitive in identifying skull fractures.
  - ☐ No particular skull fracture pattern specifically suggests abuse.
  - ☐ Fractures may be difficult to diagnose in the presence of unfused sutures in young patients.
  - ☐ Axial imaging alone is inadequate. Coronal and sagittal reformatted images must be performed.
  - ☐ Fractures are most commonly linear and have a good prognosis.
  - ☐ Diastatic fractures, i.e. those crossing suture lines, may lead to the phenomenon of a 'growing fracture' and the development of a **leptomeningeal cyst**.

☐ Careful attention should be given to the skull base, including the basilar occipital, temporal, sphenoid and ethmoid bones because these are common fracture sites in children.

Acute reporting

- Do not attempt to date injuries.
- The best indicator of abuse is an injury out of proportion to a given history.
- In children under age 2 and in selected children under age 5, advise a skeletal survey.
- Carefully document and describe fractures as these are extremely important for forensic reporting.
- When describing an injury, use terminology that is accurate and specific, clear and unequivocal.

Paediatric mesenteric and bowel injury

Typically seen in the setting of bicycle handlebar injury, child abuse or a motor vehicle accident when a lap belt is positioned too high over the abdomen. Symptoms of bowel injury are often clinically subtle.

What to look for on CT

- *Lap belt ecchymosis:* This is shown as soft tissue stranding in the subcutaneous tissues of the mid-abdomen.
- Unexplained peritoneal fluid. Free fluid in the absence of a recognizable solid organ injury may be the only sign.
- Abnormal bowel wall enhancement, bowel wall thickening (>2–3 mm), mural haematoma or bowel wall disruption.
- Stranding within the mesentery or a **sentinal clot** – high-density haematoma in the mesentery adjacent to site of bowel injury
- Pneumoperitoneum – use wide windows rather than lung windows or the invert function on the PACS workstation to detect free gas.
- Look for associated retroperitoneal injury such as to pancreas.
- Look for vascular abnormalities such as mesenteric pseudoaneurysm or contrast extravasation.
- Look for associated spinal injury, such as a Chance fracture.

Interventional aspects

In the case of solid organ injury, the patient's clinical status primarily determines whether management will be surgical or conservative. With hollow viscus injury, most children will proceed to surgery. When active extravasation or mesenteric pseudoaneurysm is identified, prompt evaluation with angiography should follow.

Acute reporting

- Record free intraperitoneal gas, bowel wall defects and focal bowel wall thickening as these usually indicate the need for surgical intervention.
- When an isolated duodenal haematoma is found, ensure that the history adequately explains the mechanism of injury as these can be seen in non-accidental trauma.

Hypoperfusion complex

Severe hypovolaemic shock in children may be masked at initial presentation, and impending cardiorespiratory failure may be first diagnosed on CT. Children will maintain their systolic blood pressure until very late in the clinical course. Tachycardia and other signs of decreased distal perfusion, such as cool extremities, delayed capillary refill and thready distal pulses, are better markers of haemodynamic instability. This phenomenon of normotension despite significant volume loss reflects the unique paediatric cardiovascular physiology. Differential vasospasm maintains perfusion to vital organs with relative underperfusion of other relatively more expendable anatomy, such as the splanchnic circulation. This process of visceral hypoperfusion can be visualized on abdominal CT and it may be the radiologist who makes the diagnosis in time to initiate life-saving resuscitation.

Conventional teaching generally reserves CT for those patients who are felt to be haemodynamically stable. Therefore, children deemed clinically stable despite being on the verge of cardiovascular collapse may be referred to CT before decompensated shock is apparent. Adults tend to descend into decompensated shock in a more gradual manner that is likely to be recognized clinically in time to intervene.

What to look for on CT

- The aorta will appear small because of vasospasm. Venous changes reflect hypovolaemia.
- The inferior vena cava, superior mesenteric vein and renal veins are diminutive.
- Haemoperitoneum will be recognized by high-density peritoneal fluid which typically will form dependent layers.

- The splanchnic circulation is preferentially sacrificed. The underperfused bowel dilates and becomes fluid filled. Mural oedema develops, along with avid mural enhancement.
- The spleen, kidneys and pancreas may show reduced enhancement as part of the compensatory shut down mechanism.
- The adrenal glands secrete epinephrine and norepinephrine, reflecting increased sympathetic tone, which leads to intense adrenal enhancement.

Acute reporting

- ***Immediately alert the clinical team of your findings:*** This can be life-saving. Once a child enters decompensated shock, cardiac arrest can rapidly follow and children who undergo cardiac arrest have a very poor chance of intact neurological survival.

Recommended reading

Bechtel K, Stoessel K, Leventhal JM, et al. Characteristics that distinguish accidental from abusive injury in hospitalized young children with head trauma. *Pediatrics* 2004;**114**:165–8.

Bulas DI, Fitz CR, Johnson DL. Traumatic atlanto-occipital dislocation in children. *Radiology* 1993;**188**:155–8.

Ruess L, Sivit CJ, Eichelberger MR, Gotschall CS, Taylor GA. Blunt abdominal trauma in children: impact of CT on operative and nonoperative management. *AJR Am J Roentgenol* 1997;**169**:1011–14.

Sivit CJ, Ingram JD, Taylor GA, et al. Posttraumatic shock in children: CT findings associated with hemodynamic instability. *Radiology* 1992;**182**:723–6.

Strouse PJ, Close BJ, Marshall KW, Cywes R. CT of bowel and mesenteric trauma in children. *Radiographics* 1999;**19**:1237–50.

Taylor GA, Fallat ME, Eichelberger MR. Hypovolemic shock in children: abdominal CT manifestations. *Radiology* 1987;**164**:479–81.

Viccellio P, Simon H, Pressman BD, et al. A prospective multicenter study of cervical spine injury in children. *Pediatrics* 2001;**108**:E20.

Neurotrauma in adults

Base of skull fracture

Summary

Protocol: Non-contrast examination with thin sections.

What to look for: Fracture lines, opacified sinuses and mastoid air cells.

Report: Describe each fracture looking for complications such as vascular injury or potential hearing compromise.

Base of skull fractures are potentially dangerous injuries and are often missed. They are known to occur in about 20% of all head injuries.

Protocol and technique

Contrast enhancement: Non-contrast examination. If a potential injury to vascular structures is suspected, a CT angiogram should be performed.

Slice collimation: Thin 0.625 mm sections with multiplanar reformats.

What to look for on CT

- Air/fluid levels or opacification of the sinuses (especially the sphenoid) is a good indicator of an occult base of skull injury.
- Pneumocephalus is another good indicator of base of skull fracture.
- Look for longitudinal or transverse fractures through the sphenoid sinus. If the fracture line traverses any foramen carrying a blood vessel, CT angiography is required.
- Look for any atlanto-occipital dissociation, which is strongly associated with fractures of the occipital condyle.
- Are the mastoid air cells well aerated? Is there a fracture through the petrous pyramid of the temporal bone?

Acute reporting

- Describe each fracture line, note any associated complication and advise if any further imaging is required.

Recommended reading

Rogers LF. Radiology of Skeletal Trauma, 3rd edn, vol 1. Edinburgh: Churchill Livingstone, 2001.

Diffuse axonal injury

Summary

Protocol: Non-contrast imaging.

What to look for: Petechial haemorrhage.

Report: Extent and multiplicity of lesions; secondary signs.

Diffuse axonal injury (DAI) is the result of trauma-induced shearing forces caused by sudden acceleration and deceleration movements affecting the grey–white interfaces of the brain parenchyma and blood vessels. The classical presentation is loss of consciousness at ictus. As such it represents severe closed head injury and detection on early imaging is crucial to guide management. CT may be normal or only show subtle abnormalities, and detection requires a high index of suspicion. The patient's history and clinical status (often much worse than the CT findings) should be taken into account and repeat CT imaging or MRI should be an early consideration.

Protocol and technique

Contrast enhancement: Non-contrast examination.

Slice collimation: 2.5 mm or less

What to look for on CT

- CT may be entirely normal or just reveal diffuse cerebral swelling.
- Evaluate those specific sites where foci of petechial haemorrhage may be identified; lobar white matter at the grey–white interface (most commonly the frontotemporal region), the corpus callosum (typically posterior body), brain stem (dorsolateral aspect), basal ganglia and internal capsule.
- Subarachnoid haemorrhage may accompany DAI.
- Delayed scanning should be considered if the early scan is normal and the clinical suspicion for DAI remains high.

Differential diagnosis

Cortical contusions can sometimes mimic diffuse axonal injury. These appear as foci of increased density, typically in the temporal lobe close to the dural lining or the frontal lobe convexity. They may be associated with local mass effect. Always look for a contre coup injury, typically at the inferior surface of the frontal and temporal lobes.

Acute reporting

- Comment on extent, multiplicity and location of any high-density lesions.
- Comment on any cerebral swelling.
- If the study is normal, suggest repeat CT or consider MRI.

Recommended reading

Gentry LR, Godersky JC, Thompson B, Dunn VD. Prospective comparative study of intermediate-field MR and CT in the evaluation of closed head trauma. *AJR Am J Roentgenol* 1988;**150**:673–82.

Toyama Y, Kobayashi T, Nishiyama Y, Satoh K, Ohkawa M, Seki K. CT for acute stage of closed head injury. *Radiat Med* 2005;**23**:309–16.

4 Abdomen and Pelvis

Acute appendicitis

Summary

Protocol: Oral and intravenous (IV) contrast, portal venous phase imaging.

What to look for: Dilated thick-walled appendix, an appendicolith, peri-appendiceal inflammatory changes, perforation.

Report: Confirm or exclude diagnosis of acute appendicitis; note extent of secondary inflammatory changes and any complications; suggest differential diagnosis.

Acute appendicitis remains the commonest cause of an acute surgical abdomen and is not uncommonly found while imaging for other suspected acute abdominal problems. The surgical adage that acute appendicitis should never be considered lower than number two in any differential diagnosis of the acute abdomen applies equally to radiological evaluation. In young female patients, ultrasound is the preferred initial imaging test as the presentation of acute tubo-ovarian pathologies can closely mimic appendicitis. Graded compression and colour flow Doppler ultrasound techniques have high diagnostic accuracy in experienced hands.

Protocol and technique

Contrast enhancement:
- **Oral contrast:** Positive contrast is preferred with full abdominal and pelvic coverage. This helps the radiologist distinguish enteric from extraenteric pathology. Some centres include rectal contrast delivery as part of the standard acute appendicitis protocol to improve their evaluation of the right iliac fossa anatomy and any periappendiceal complication.
- **IV contrast:** 100 ml contrast at 3 ml/s with single-phase, portal venous image acquisition.

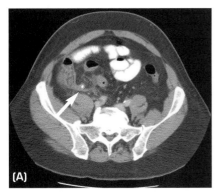

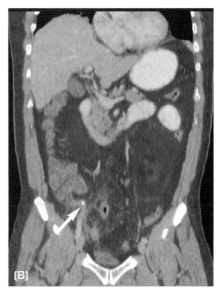

Figure 4.1: Acute appendicitis.
Right iliac fossa pain. Both axial and coronal CT images demonstrate a dilated fluid-filled appendix with surrounding inflammatory changes. Arrows show appendicolith within inflamed appendix.

Slice collimation: 2.5–5 mm axial reconstruction with coronal and sagittal reformats as required.

What to look for on CT

- A dilated (>6 mm) and thick walled appendix (Fig. 4.1): 6 mm is the commonly quoted upper limit of normal but some authors consider calibres of up to 10 mm as normal. A mildly dilated appendix with no associated inflammatory changes is an unlikely cause of the patient's abdominal pain. Appendiceal wall thickening is influenced by the degree of luminal fluid distension.
- An appendicolith. The presence of an appendicolith supports the diagnosis of acute appendicitis but is not by itself diagnostic.
- Periappendiceal inflammatory change and adjacent fascial plane thickening. Differentiate between local peritonitic change and more generalized peritonitis found in severe cases (Fig. 4.2).
- Typically, there is an absence of oral contrast within the appendix lumen even when the small bowel is well opacified with contrast.
- Periappendiceal abscess formation (Fig. 4.3).
- Inflammation can track in a cephalad direction to involve the bare area of the liver, particularly in children. Hepatic abscess is another recognized complication.
- Appendiceal perforation. CT findings suggestive of a perforated appendix include:

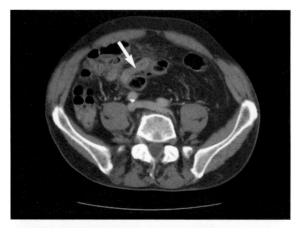

Figure 4.2: Acute appendicitis. Dilated appendix with tip extending to the midline of the lower abdomen (arrow). Note dirty fat anterior to the dilated appendix, contrasting with normal fat densities elsewhere in the section.

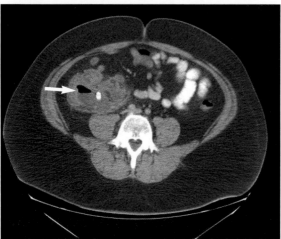

Figure 4.3: Complicated appendicitis. An appendicular abscess with air–fluid level (arrow) and adjacent appendicolith.

- ☐ An appendicolith seen *outside* the appendix.
- ☐ A focal defect in the wall of the appendix.
- ☐ Extraluminal air adjacent to the appendix. Depending on the duration of the illness, air may be detected at some distance from the appendix.
- ☐ Periappendiceal fluid collection.
- ☐ Rarely septic emboli may complicate acute appendicitis leading to superior mesenteric/portal vein thrombosis and portal pyaemia.

Interventional aspects: drainage of an appendiceal abscess

Abscess drainage should only be attempted when a well-defined periappendiceal collection measuring over 3 cm is present and there is a safe route of access for drainage.

> ## Points to remember
>
> - Patients with mild *isolated* dilatation of the appendix (<10 mm) without any other inflammatory change are unlikely to have appendicitis.
> - Fewer than 30% of patients with an identifiable *normal* appendix surrounded by inflammatory stranding or fluid will have appendicitis.
> - Do not forget the variants:
>   - Distal or tip appendicitis where the proximal appendiceal segment is normal.
>   - Recurrent or chronic appendicitis, which have reported incidences of 10% and 1%, respectively.
>   - Stump appendicitis.
> - Always try and ensure the patient has an appendix in situ before offering a diagnosis of acute appendicitis, but do not forget the possibility of stump appendicitis which appears to be commoner post laparoscopic appendicectomy if the stump has not been adequately buried.

Differential diagnosis

Segmental omental infarction (Fig. 4.4)

This is a close mimic of acute appendicitis, typically presenting with an acute onset of right iliac fossa pain. Trauma or thrombosis of the omental venous drainage leads to this complication.

What to look for on CT:
- Try and identify a normal appendix and a normal terminal ileum in the first instance.
- Look for a focal area of increased fatty density located lateral to the right colon that typically exerts mass effect on the adjacent bowel.
- Patients may exhibit focal tenderness on direct palpation over the area of CT abnormality.
- Omental infarction may be encountered following intra-abdominal surgery such as post hemicolectomy or oesophagogastric surgery and occasionally following a difficult hysterectomy.
- Management is conservative with no indication for surgery, assuming a confident diagnosis and supporting clinical correlation.

Epiploic appendagitis (Fig. 4.5)

This will present in a similar manner to segmental omental infarction. An epiploic appendage is a pouch-like protrusion lined by peritoneum

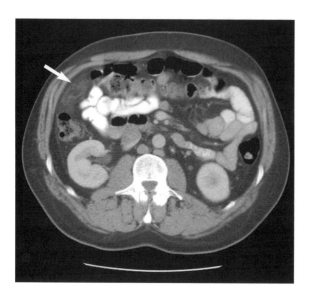

Figure 4.4: Acute segmental omental infarction. Typical finding of increased density fat with mass effect (arrow).

that arises from the serosal surface of the colon. It typically contains fat and is connected to the bowel wall by a vascular stalk. When an appendage undergoes torsion, vascular occlusion and ischaemia develop leading to acute abdominal pain. This complication occurs most commonly on the left, with left iliac fossa pain the usual presenting symptom that often mimics acute diverticulitis. Less commonly, the presentation is right sided in which circumstance acute appendicitis is often the initial clinical diagnosis. Epiploic appendagitis is a self-limiting condition and surgical intervention is not required. This, along with segmental omental infarction, are important CT diagnoses to recognize in order to prevent the patient undergoing unnecessary surgery.

What to look for on CT:
- Common sites are adjacent to the sigmoid colon, descending colon and the right hemicolon.
- Look for a fat-containing ovoid or rounded mass that can measure from 1 cm up to 5 cm in cross-section and abuts the colonic wall.
- The degree of surrounding dirty fat is variable but rarely excessive.
- An enhancing periphery and a central focal density, representing the thrombosed vessel, are typical findings.
- Patients generally respond promptly to conservative management but CT may remain abnormal for up to 6 months.

Complicated caecal malignancy

A perforated caecal malignancy can present with right iliac fossa pain and on occasion may be difficult to distinguish from the inflammatory changes of appendicitis in the acute setting.

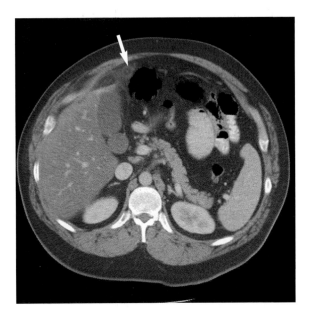

Figure 4.5: Epiploic appendagitis. Patient presented with right-sided abdominal pain. Contrast-enhanced CT shows a ring lesion with a central dot (arrow) and associated inflammatory change lying in the omentum anterior to the transverse colon.

- Look for supporting signs of malignancy elsewhere in the abdomen, such as liver metastases, locoregional lymph nodes and peritoneal tumour deposits. Pericaecal lymph nodes adjacent to a focal area of caecal wall thickening are more commonly seen in patients with cancer than in those with diverticulitis.
- A stratified enhancement pattern in a thickened segment of bowel wall virtually excludes malignancy.
- Fat stranding out of proportion to the degree of wall thickening is more typical of inflammatory conditions than malignancy.

Acute gynaecological pathology

Caecal diverticulitis

Acute presentation Crohn's disease

Complicated Meckel's diverticulum

Acute reporting

- Confirm or exclude a diagnosis of acute appendicitis. Describe associated inflammatory changes and any complications.
- If a diagnosis is not made, offer a reasonable differential keeping in mind the patient's age and clinical presentation.
- When appropriate, discuss merits of imaging guided intervention as alternative to a surgical procedure with referring clinician.

Recommended reading

Birnbaum BA, Wilson SR. Appendicitis at the millennium. *Radiology* 2000;**215**:337–48.

Hoeffel C, Crema MD, Belkacem A, Azizi L, Lewin M, Arrivé L, Tubiana JM. Multi-detector row CT: spectrum of diseases involving the ileocecal area. *Radiographics* 2006;**26**:1373–90.

Singh AK, Gervais DA, Hahn PF, Sagar P, Mueller PR, Novelline RA. Acute epiploic appendagitis and its mimics. *Radiographics* 2005;**25**:1521–34.

Acute cholecystitis

Summary

Protocol: Oral and IV contrast. Image in portal venous phase.

Look for: Gallstones, gallbladder wall thickening, pericholecystic oedema. Identify biliary tree dilatation and gas in biliary tree. Look for features of emphysematous and gangrenous cholecystitis.

Report: Severity of cholecystitis, and complications such as biliary obstruction, emphysematous or gangrenous cholecystitis.

Ultrasound is generally accepted as the preferred initial imaging technique for suspected acute cholecystitis. Radionuclide imaging will confirm cystic duct obstruction but is rarely requested as part of the initial diagnostic evaluation. However, in the patient with an acute abdomen and an uncertain diagnosis, CT will usually be the imaging method chosen unless the clinical signs point to a likely right upper quadrant pathology. Multidetector CT (MDCT) has a high sensitivity and specificity in the diagnosis of acute cholecystitis (up to 95%).

Protocol and technique

Contrast enhancement:

- **Oral contrast:** Positive contrast preferred with an abdominal volume. Oral contrast is especially useful to clarify the anatomy around the duodenal sweep.
- **IV contrast:** In most acute situations, the gallbladder will be assessed as part of a survey study of the abdomen and pelvis. Images should be acquired in the portal venous phase after 100 ml of contrast delivered at 3 ml/s.

Slice collimation: 2.5–5 mm axial reconstruction.

What to look for on CT

Calculus cholecystitis

- Localized inflammatory change centred on the right upper quadrant, including gallbladder wall thickening (>3 mm), pericholecystic inflammation and fluid.
- Gallstones will only be visible in approximately 50% of CT examinations (Figs 4.6, 4.7).
- Inflammatory changes may influence neighbouring anatomy. The adjacent liver parenchyma can display focal hyperenhancement, and mural thickening of the hepatic flexure of the colon may be present. This finding can lead to an alternative diagnosis such as acute diverticulitis being considered. The hepatic flexure is an uncommon site for acute diverticulitis.

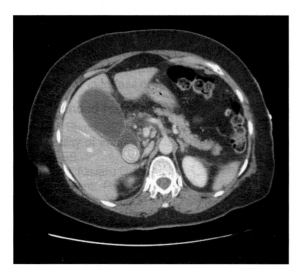

Figure 4.6: Acute cholecystitis.
Laminated gallstone in the neck of a distended gallbladder. Note inflammatory changes within fat between the gallbladder and the posterior aspect of the left liver.

Acalculus cholecystitis

- Accounts for 5–10% of all cases of acute cholecystitis and is associated with a significantly higher morbidity and mortality. It is more commonly found in patients with severe intercurrent illness (particularly intensive care patients) and in patients on total parenteral nutrition.
- This is an almost impossible CT diagnosis due to gallstones not being visible in half the cases of the much commoner calculus cholecystitis. Ultrasound will be required to differentiate between the two conditions. Nevertheless, it is important to consider this diagnosis in patient groups with an increased risk, e.g. intensive care patients.
- CT findings are similar to those found in calculus cholecystitis with mural thickening and pericholecystic fluid being typical features.

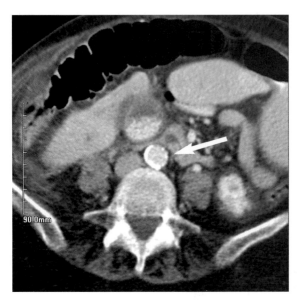

Figure 4.7: Acute cholecystitis and choledocholithiasis. Thick-walled gallbladder containing multiple calculi. Pericholecystic fluid and stones within the common bile duct. In this elderly patient, the gallbladder lies towards the midline of the abdomen with the pancreatic head lying to the left of the midline. These features gave a confusing clinical picture.

- There is an increased incidence of gangrenous change and subsequent perforation with acalculus cholecystitis.

Complications of acute cholecystitis

- **Gallbladder empyema:** Stagnation of infected bile leads to frank pus accumulating within the gallbladder lumen. This potential complication occurs with both calculus and acalculus cholecystitis and, if the pressure within the gallbladder is not relieved, gangrene, perforation and generalized sepsis can develop. An empyema may be difficult to differentiate from a non-infected bile-containing gallbladder in otherwise uncomplicated acute cholecystitis. Clinical correlation will be required but ultrasound or CT-guided aspiration will be necessary to confirm the diagnosis.

- **Emphysematous cholecystitis:** This complication is rare (1% of all cases of acute cholecystitis), is usually found in elderly diabetic patients and has a male preponderance. The mortality rate is high at 15–20%, with *Clostridium welchii* being the commonest causative organism. CT features include gas in the gallbladder wall or gallbladder lumen. Gas may occasionally be found in the pericholecystic tissues.

- **Gangrenous cholecystitis:** Gangrenous or necrotizing cholecystitis is a severe form of acute cholecystitis characterized by increased gallbladder distension and marked thickening of the gallbladder wall leading to ischaemic necrosis and perforation. The diagnosis is often only made at surgery, but certain CT features should alert the radiologist to the possibility of this diagnosis (Fig. 4.8):

☐ Mural irregularity and mural striation (alternating high- and low-density layers).
☐ Increased gallbladder luminal distension.
☐ Absence of an enhancing gallbladder wall.
☐ Intraluminal 'membranes' (usually recognized as linear foci of high density).

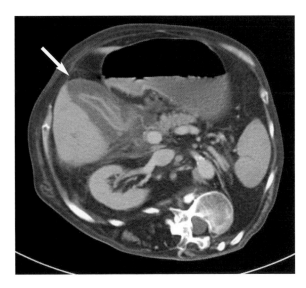

Figure 4.8: Gangrenous cholecystitis. Gross gallbladder mural thickening (arrow) should always suggest the possibility of gangrenous cholecystitis.

■ *Gallbladder perforation:* Excessive pericholecystic fluid should alert the radiologist to the possibility of gallbladder perforation. Leaked bile may also track down the right paracolic gutter as a localized extension of the pericholecystic change, rather than as part of a more generalized ascites. Identifying a gallbladder wall defect, though uncommonly seen, confirms the diagnosis.
■ *Abscess formation:* Differentiating pericholecystic abscess from simple pericholecystic fluid can be difficult, and typically the diagnosis will only be made following percutaneous aspiration. As with abscesses elsewhere in the abdominal cavity, they may exhibit abnormal wall enhancement, a minority contain gas, and mass affect may be noted on neighbouring structures.
■ *Biliary tree dilatation:* When biliary tree dilatation is present, attempt to identify the level of obstruction. Distal bile duct compromise is usually due to a stone in the common bile duct. Subtle density differences are frequently seen in the distal common bile duct on CT and a firm diagnosis of choledocholithiasis may be difficult unless an obvious calculus is present. Multiplanar reformatted images in the coronal plane can be helpful. More proximal compromise might reflect a Mirizzi situation where the extrahepatic biliary tree is compromised

by a calculus in the adjacent cystic duct. If there is diagnostic doubt as to whether duct stones are present, magnetic resonance cholangiopancreatography (MRCP) should be arranged at the earliest opportunity.

Differential diagnosis

- A confident diagnosis of acute cholecystitis can be made when characteristic clinical and imaging findings are present. The main differential includes acute pancreatitis, upper gastrointestinal perforation and acute appendicitis.
- Remember there are numerous causes of gallbladder wall thickening unrelated to acute gallbladder inflammation, including ascites, hypoproteinaemia and heart failure.
- Causes of gas in the biliary tree include post biliary intervention such as endoscopic retrograde cholangiopancreatography (ERCP) and sphincterotomy, biliary–enteric fistula formation and cholangitis with gas-forming organisms.

Interventional aspects: imaging-guided drainage of empyema/pericholecystic abscess

Percutaneous drainage under ultrasound or CT guidance can be life-saving, particularly in the elderly when emergency surgical intervention might be considered too risky. As always, close clinicoradiological liaison is required. Look for a safe route of entry. Whether a transhepatic or non-transhepatic route is chosen is down to local preference and clotting status.

Acute reporting

- Confirm the diagnosis of cholecystitis.
- Look for gallstones and duct stones.
- Assess the degree of gallbladder distension and look for luminal gas.
- Evaluate mural changes looking for irregular thickening, mural striation, loss of mural enhancement and mural gas.
- Assess the pericholecystic changes, particularly the extent of pericholecystic fluid and any suspected abscess formation.
- When prominent mural thickening is accompanied by increased luminal distension, always consider the possibility of gangrenous cholecystitis.

Recommended reading

Alterman DD, Hocbsztein JG. Computed tomography in acute cholecystitis. *Emerg Radiol* 1996;**3**:25–9.

Bennett GL, Rusinek H, Lisi V, et al. CT findings in acute gangrenous chole-cystitis. *AJR Am J Roentgenol* 2002;**178**:275–81.

Acute pancreatitis

Summary

Protocol: Oral and IV contrast. Three-phase study: unenhanced, interstitial and portal venous phases.

Look for: Haemorrhage, pancreatic and biliary calcification on unenhanced phase; on post contrast phases, pancreatic necrosis; peri-pancreatic inflammatory changes and fluid collections; vascular complications.

Report: Severity of pancreatitis – necrotizing or interstitial, extent of extrapancreatic changes. Record complications and suggest possible aetiology.

The diagnosis of acute pancreatitis is based on clinical and biochemical assessment. The role of imaging is to confirm the diagnosis when there is clinical uncertainty, to assess the severity of the attack, and identify any complications. In the acute situation, CT is best suited to provide this information.

Protocol and technique

Contrast enhancement:

- **Oral contrast:** Oral contrast is advisable to delineate the bowel anatomy and differentiate extraenteric fluid from normal gastric and small bowel content. Abdominal coverage with positive or negative contrast agents. Patients who are on a nil-by-mouth regimen may benefit from the contrast being delivered via a nasogastric tube.
- **Intravenous contrast:** A three-phase protocol is typically used for the initial diagnostic scan. The protocol may be modified for any follow-up imaging depending on the clinical status.
  - ☐ **Non-contrast phase:** Commence imaging at lung bases and continue through the pancreatic bed. This will demonstrate pancreatic and biliary calcification as well as any acute haemorrhagic change within the pancreatic parenchyma and in the extrapancreatic tissues. Whether completion coverage of the extrapancreatic inflammatory changes is performed during this phase or left until the portal venous phase is down to local preference. At least for the initial diagnostic study, complete abdominal and pelvic coverage is advisable at some stage of the protocol to cover all sites of potential

extrapancreatic inflammatory spread. Full chest coverage is generally not required unless initial imaging reveals unexpected intrathoracic extension of the inflammatory process.

☐ ***Post IV contrast:*** Interstitial phase imaging (a little later than arterial phase, at approximately 40 seconds post onset of injection) optimizes assessment of pancreatic parenchymal enhancement and therefore is the ideal phase to establish whether parenchymal necrosis is present or absent. Arterial complications will also be detected during this phase, whereas venous problems will be best appreciated during the portal venous phase.

Slice reconstruction: 5 mm sections for non-contrast series, 2.5 mm for interstitial phase, and 2.5–5 mm for portal venous phase.

What to look for on CT?

Imaging may be entirely normal in cases of mild and early pancreatitis.

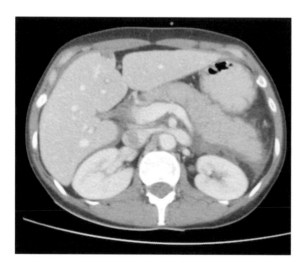

Figure 4.9: Acute interstitial pancreatitis. The pancreas is swollen with peripancreatic inflammatory fluid seen around the tail.

Pancreatic assessment

■ On the non-contrast images, look for **calcification** and signs of recent **haemorrhage.**

■ Identify focal or diffuse **enlargement** of the pancreas (Fig. 4.9).

■ Establish whether parenchymal **necrosis** is present and indicate its extent. Necrosis is defined as an area of non-enhancement or significantly reduced parenchymal enhancement measuring 3 cm or greater (Figs 4.10, 4.11). Diagnose by using the region of interest cursor and compare the pre- and post-contrast images. Enhancement of less than 30 Hounsfield Units (HU) will indicate necrosis. Hounsfield Units are a measure of tissue density on CT and can be indicated as a mouse cursor value as the reader scrolls across the image or by selecting a specific region of interest calculation. A more practical approach is to simply perform an eyeball comparison of pancreatic parenchymal enhancement with that of adjacent spleen. **Do not compare with liver as fatty change within the liver will be a common finding in acute pancreatitis and can lead to spurious conclusions.** Remember also that if CT is performed too early in an attack of acute pancreatitis, necrosis may not yet be established and a false diagnosis of interstitial pancreatitis may result. Scanning less than 48 hours into an attack is unhelpful from the necrosis aspect, but earlier than ideal scanning may be required if there is diagnostic doubt in a patient with an acute abdomen.

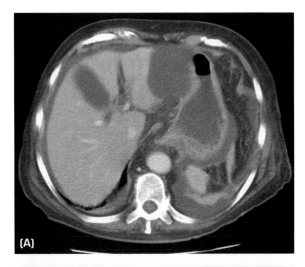

(A)

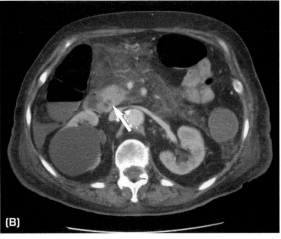

(B)

Figure 4.10: Acute necrotizing gall stone pancreatitis. (A) A left pleural effusion, ascites, perihepatic and perigastric fluid collections. A section of normal pancreatic tail enhancement seen behind stomach.
(B) Parenchymal necrosis of the neck and proximal body of the pancreas with normal enhancement of the head. Note the extrapancreatic inflammatory changes involving the mesentery and retroperitoneum. Focal density in the distal common bile duct (arrow) represents a duct calculus.

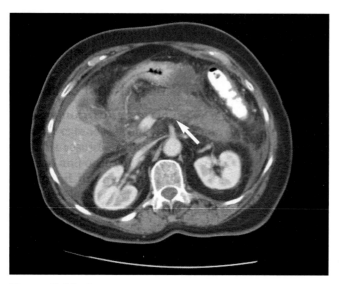

Figure 4.11: Severe acute necrotizing pancreatitis. On this section, global parenchymal necrosis. The variation in parenchymal density reflects variable degrees of liquifaction. On other sections, the inferior aspect of the pancreatic head was viable but the degree of overall parenchymal necrosis was in excess of 80%. Note the splenic vein is thrombosed (arrow). Extensive extrapancreatic inflammatory changes with retroperitoneal fluid, ascites and a fluid collection forming behind stomach. Multiple gallstones are also present, indicating the likely aetiology for this acute attack.

- Peripancreatic necrosis will show as a rind of low-density soft tissue, picture framing the pancreatic contour.

Extrapancreatic assessment

- Identify **inflammatory exudate** in the peripancreatic tissues, other retroperitoneal spaces and the peritoneal cavity. Note secondary effects on adjacent anatomy which can include prominent mural thickening of stomach, small bowel and colon, which can lead to diagnostic confusion.
- Look for thickening and reduced clarity of the retroperitoneal fascial planes.
- *Acute fluid collection, abscess and ascites:* Acute fluid collections are characterized by pockets of fluid density that are contained and shaped by the surrounding anatomy. They tend to occur early in the attack but with time, usually 4–6 weeks, a capsule of non-epithelialized granulation tissue can develop around persisting collections, which is a characteristic feature of an **acute pseudocyst** (Fig. 4.12).

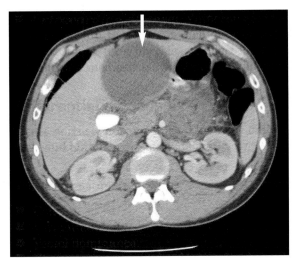

Figure 4.12: Acute Pancreatic pseudocysts – example of encapsulated mature fluid collection (arrow) in a patient who had a recent attack of acute pancreatitis.

Abscess formation is typically a late complication and percutaneous aspiration may be required to differentiate infection from a non-infected simple fluid collection (see later). Gas will be evident in only the minority of abscesses (Fig. 4.13). Abscesses also differ from simple fluid collections by typically displaying mass effect on the surrounding anatomy. Ascites is a common finding in acute pancreatitis and indicates a further adverse prognostic factor in most scoring systems.

- *Pleural effusion:* Left-sided effusions are commoner than right-sided, but bilateral changes are often present. An absence of pleural fluid in a severe attack would be an unusual finding.
- Identify **vascular** complications – splenic vein thrombosis, less commonly portal vein thrombosis, and pseudoaneurysm formation. Carefully identify all areas of vascular enhancement and establish whether these correspond to normal vascular anatomy. The enhancement characteristics of a pseudoaneurysm will mirror adjacent normal vessels, so compare the degree of enhancement and contrast wash out with the aorta or superior mesenteric artery. Contrast extravasation will show persisting or increased enhancement on the later phases of imaging. Venous erosion may result in high-density change within the mesentery and this is best appreciated on the non-enhanced images. Larger haematomas may show mass effect. Do not overcall superior mesenteric vein thrombosis on interstitial phase imaging alone.
- Identify any extraenteric **gas.** Beware of potential pitfalls which include gas within a duodenal diverticulum or other adjacent segment of bowel that may have been suboptimally opacified by oral contrast. Gastrointestinal fistulae may develop secondary to acute pancreatitis but this tends to be a later complication. Always beware of iatrogenic foci of gas secondary to recent surgical or interventional procedures.

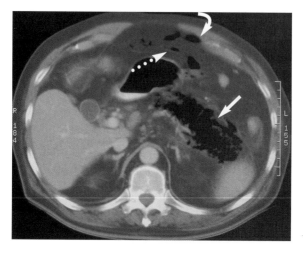

Figure 4.13: Complicated pancreatitis. Infected parenchymal necrosis with gas densities replacing the normal parenchyma (arrow). Note also the presence of free intraperitoneal gas (curved arrow), as well as gas located within the mesenteric vein branches (dotted arrow).

- Always remember that **bowel ischaemia** can develop as a complication of acute pancreatitis. This is a difficult clinical diagnosis as metabolic acidosis may be a part of the multiorgan failure picture found with severe pancreatitis. Gastrointestinal mural thickening, which may be marked and is typically of low density, is a common finding irrespective of whether ischaemia is present or absent. Nevertheless, ischaemia must be considered, particularly when there is unexplained clinical deterioration or increasing acidosis. Look for mural haemorrhage on the non-contrast images, and increased or absent mural enhancement on the post-contrast series.

Suggest a likely aetiology

- Look for gallstones, bile duct calculi or biliary dilatation. Generally, ultrasound will be required to confirm or exclude biliary disease and current guidelines state that a minimum of two negative ultrasound studies are required before biliary disease is discounted as a likely cause. If biliary dilatation is present, MRCP will be required to confirm or exclude duct calculi.
- Look for **pancreatic calcification** indicating acute on chronic pancreatitis.
- Identify **fatty change** in liver that might indicate alcohol abuse or hyperlipidaemia.
- Also look for signs of **chronic liver disease** and portal hypertension. Liver contour irregularity, altered hepatic lobar morphology with enlargement to left lobe and caudate and contraction of the right lobe, splenomegaly, varices and recanalization of the umbilical vein.
- **Anatomical variants of the pancreaticobiliary tree** are difficult to recognize on CT and MRCP will be needed at some stage if no other aetiology becomes apparent.

- *Autoimmune pancreatitis:* Always consider when no other precipitating cause is apparent as this condition responds to steroid therapy. An attack may lead to focal or generalized pancreatitis. A thin rind of soft tissue may surround the swollen pancreas with little other evidence of peripancreatic inflammation. The pancreatic parenchyma may display a lattice-work or herring bone enhancement pattern. Look for recognized extrapancreatic associations, such as focal renal defects and retroperitoneal lymphadenopathy. A demonstration of elevated serum immunoglobulin levels, notably IgG4, will confirm autoimmune pancreatitis.

Differential diagnosis

There is really no tenable differential diagnosis when the classical imaging findings of acute pancreatitis are present and a confident imaging-based diagnosis should be made in most cases, unless imaging occurs too early in the disease process.

The main clinical differential is acute cholecystitis and upper gastrointestinal perforation.

Interventional aspects: CT-guided drainage of collections

Remember that simple fluid, pus and necrosis can appear identical on CT, each displaying comparable low attenuation CT numbers. CT is extremely poor at characterizing the internal characteristics of fluid collections. What may appear to be simple fluid on CT may be predominantly solid on other imaging such as ultrasound or MRI. **It is therefore imperative to avoid the risk of introducing infection into a sterile environment by inappropriate or misguided percutaneous aspiration or drainage.** The prognosis for infected necrosis is significantly worse than that of sterile necrosis. Always discuss intervention with the referring clinician before any decision is made. If aspiration/drainage is indicated on clinical grounds, and access is difficult, a transgastric approach is perfectly acceptable and is often preferable to the direct route. Never traverse the colon. Very rarely, a transhepatic approach can be used, assuming there is no other means of safe access.

A simple diagnostic aspiration may be all that is required. If no pus is found, the view may be taken to avoid catheter placement until culture results are available. Not infrequently, multiple catheter placements will be required depending on the patient's clinical status and extent of extrapancreatic inflammatory change. It is always worth discussing potential future management options before placing a drainage catheter. If percutaneous necrosectomy is being considered, then ideally the catheter should be placed using a left posterolateral approach, assuming a safe route of access is available that the avoids spleen and colon.

Acute reporting

The CT findings contribute to the overall staging of disease severity. It is therefore important to record all abnormalities that have a prognostic significance. A number of pancreatic scoring systems are well documented in the literature, but in the UK, these have not been widely incorporated into day-to-day routine reporting practice.

- Confirm the diagnosis, indicate degree of severity and describe any complications.
- Differentiate between acute interstitial pancreatitis and acute necrotizing pancreatitis.
- When necrosis is present, give a guestimated percentage of parenchymal loss involved. A useful guide would be less than one-third, between one-third and one-half, and greater than 50% as a ball park indication.
- Record the presence and absence of vascular complications. Discuss any vascular malformations or evidence of acute bleeding with the referring clinician and interventional radiologist.

When describing extrapancreatic fluid collections try to use the following terms:

- *Acute fluid collection:* These occur early in the course of acute pancreatitis and are located in or near the pancreas. They always lack a definable wall and are contained by whatever anatomical structures they come in contact with.
- *Acute pseudocyst:* This is a collection of pancreatic juices enclosed by a non-epithelialized wall. By definition, these take at least 4 weeks to develop.
- *Pancreatic abscess:* A circumscribed collection of pus, typically lying close to the pancreas, which contains little or no necrosis. These tend to occur later in the illness.

Recommended reading

Alhajeri A, Erwin S. Acute pancreatitis: value and impact of CT severity index. *Abdom Imaging* 2008;**33**:18–20.

Balthazar EJ. Acute pancreatitis: assessment of severity with clinical and CT evaluation. *Radiology* 2002;**223**:603–13.

Morgan DE. Imaging of acute pancreatitis and its complications. *Clin Gastroenterol Hepatol* 2008;**6**:1077–85.

Acute diverticulitis

Summary

Protocol: Oral and IV contrast. Image in portal venous phase.

What to look for: Diverticulosis, perienteric inflammatory changes, associated abscess, fistula, perforation with extra-luminal and portal venous gas.

Report: Extent and severity of diverticulitis and any complications.

The term diverticulosis refers to the presence of sac-like outpouchings (diverticula) arising from the bowel wall, which may be filled with air, faeces or oral contrast. Diverticula can be found throughout the gastrointestinal tract but occur most frequently in the sigmoid colon. Diverticulitis results from obstruction to the neck of a diverticulum with subsequent microperforation leading to pericolonic inflammation. The incidence of diverticulosis increases with age, with >80% of the population older than 85 years said to be affected. With changes in dietary patterns, diverticular disease and its complications are increasingly recognized in much younger age groups. CT is reported to be highly sensitive and specific in the diagnosis of diverticulitis and its complications.

Protocol and technique

Contrast enhancement:

- ***Oral contrast:*** Positive contrast with a full abdominal and pelvic volume. The urinary bladder should be full. Oral contrast delineates the small bowel anatomy and helps differentiate extraenteric pathology from normal and abnormal bowel. Rectal contrast would not be considered a routine requirement.
- ***IV contrast:*** 100 ml of iodinated contrast at 3 ml/s with images acquired during the portal venous phase.

Slice collimation: 2.5–5 mm. Coverage should include the abdomen and pelvis from the diaphragm down to the symphysis pubis.

What to look for on CT

- Confirm the presence of diverticula and associated mural thickening. Inflamed colon will typically display increased mural enhancement when compared to non-inflamed colon. Depending on the degree of

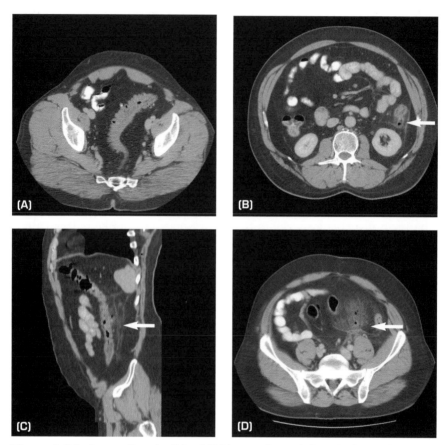

Figure 4.14: Acute diverticulitis: **(A)** Uncomplicated diverticulosis of the sigmoid colon with clean perienteric fat. Note high-density material in a diverticulum which is a common finding and does not indicate acute disease. (B–D) Acute descending colon diverticulitis (arrows); diverticula, dirty fat and adjacent fascial plane thickening establish the diagnosis. Always consider the possibility of dual pathology in areas of severe diverticular disease. Although often impossible to categorically exclude coexisting malignancy, the presence of associated lymphadenopathy or liver metastases will suggest likely dual pathology.

mural thickening, there may be associated compromise to the colonic lumen which can lead to large bowel obstruction.

- Look for pericolonic inflammatory change. This can range from minor 'dirty fat' to an extensive inflammatory mass with pockets of fluid and abscess formation (Figs 4.14, 4.15).
- Identify the common complications of acute diverticulitis:
  - **Pericolic abscess:** A localized collection of high fluid or low-density soft tissue usually with an enhancing wall that may or may not

contain gas. Abscesses tend to exert mass effect on the surrounding anatomy (Fig. 4.16).

☐ **Fistula formation:** Look for fistulous extension into adjacent structures such as the urinary bladder, iliopsoas muscle or sacroiliac joint. Fistulae appear as linear structures of gas or fluid density that arise from the inflamed segment of bowel and extend into adjacent organs, bowel loops or skin surface. Focal bladder wall thickening in the setting of severe sigmoid diverticulitis may be an early sign of impending fistula formation. Air in the urinary bladder without a supporting history of recent instrumentation will usually indicate a colovesical fistula (Fig. 4.17).

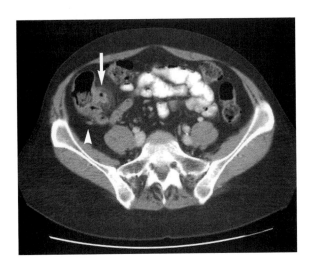

Figure 4.15: Caecal diverticulitis (arrow). The clinical presentation will usually be identical to acute appendicitis. Look for diverticula, signs of acute inflammation and a normal appendix (arrowhead).

☐ **Perforation:** Most diverticula develop along the mesenteric border of the colon and extraluminal gas is usually seen between the leaves of the sigmoid mesocolon. In acute diverticulitis, extraluminal gas is typically confined to the immediate pericolonic tissues, but on occasion can lead to a generalized pneumoperitoneum (Fig. 4.16). This may be found when patients are on high-dose steroids and immunosuppression masks the initial symptoms, often leading to a delay in diagnosis. Unexplained intraperitoneal or retroperitoneal gas in the upper abdomen always requires the exclusion of pelvic pathology. Established peritonitis will result in diffuse or patchy dirty peritoneal fat, variable thickening of the peritoneal reflections, and scattered pockets of intraperitoneal fluid.

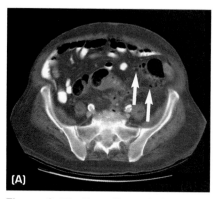
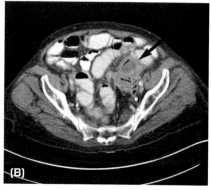

Figure 4.16: Complicated diverticulitis. (A) Perforated diverticulitis with foci of extraenteric gas within the mesentery (arrows). Always try to follow the mesenteric venous branches up to the main portal vein and into liver. Look for associated liver abscess. **(B)** Perienteric diverticular abscess (arrow).

☐ **Portal pyaemia** is a recognizable complication of acute diverticulitis. Look for gas in peripheral mesenteric venous arcades, within the inferior mesenteric vein, splenic vein, and main portal vein, and into the liver. Be careful not to confuse portal venous gas with biliary tree gas. Intrahepatic portal vein gas typically accumulates *peripherally* and displays a spidery claw-like pattern, reflecting the size of the peripheral vessels. Biliary tree gas is typically seen in a more central position and can usually be traced into the common bile duct to confirm its origin.

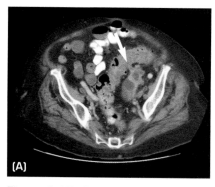
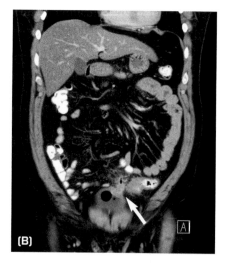

Figure 4.17: Complicated diverticulitis. (A) Colo-ovarian (arrow) and **(B)** colovesical fistulae (arrow).

Differential diagnosis

A confident diagnosis of acute diverticulitis can be made when support-ing clinical and imaging findings are present. The main differential diag-noses include:

- **Colonic cancer:** Complicated colon cancer is the main differential diagnosis and although confident differentiation between the two pathologies may be impossible in the acute setting, there may be clues which can help distinguish between the two entities. Fluid in the sig-moid mesentery with thickening of adjacent fascial planes, particularly when these track into the lower pelvis, along with engorgement of the adjacent mesenteric vessels favours inflammation over malignancy. Cancer is more likely when the colonic component is more 'mass like', perhaps with a shouldered luminal margin, along with enlarged locore-gional nodes, distant metastases or peritoneal deposits. Pericolonic inflammatory changes are typically less marked in malignancy. How-ever, in many cases sigmoidoscopy and biopsy is required to establish the diagnosis. The possibility of dual colonic pathology should always be considered in the presence of severe diverticulosis.
- **Acute appendicitis, segmental omental infarction** and **Crohn's disease** offer diagnostic alternatives to right-sided colonic diverticuli-tis. **Epiploic appendagitis** and less commonly omental infarction for left-sided diverticulitis, while **ischaemic colitis** can involve either the right or left colon. Never forget the potential for acute pan-creatic inflammatory change to track caudally, particularly on the left, and mimic primary colonic pathology.

Interventional aspects: CT-guided drainage of diverticular abscess

Where there is safe access, percutaneous drainage of a pericolonic abscess under imaging guidance offers a valuable alternative to emergency sur-gery, which most likely would result in a defunctioning stoma and the need for a second operation. Drainage may allow the elective planning of a sin-gle operative event, as well as providing a temporal window to improve a critically ill patient's clinical status prior to surgery. As with all radiologi-cal interventions, close liaison with the referring clinician is required.

Abscesses smaller than 5 cm in maximum diameter often respond favourably to intravenous antibiotics without the need for drainage. Cur-rently, some surgeons advocate a laparoscopic wash out procedure as an alternative to conventional surgery at the time of acute presentation.

Acute reporting

- Establish the diagnosis of acute diverticulitis.

- Describe its severity and location.
- Give an indication of the overall extent of diverticulosis in addition to the acute changes.
- If you cannot exclude malignancy, put that in the report. Suggesting the possibility of malignancy will benefit the referring clinician when considering the surgical options and will help in any preoperative discussions with the patient.
- Is there evidence of obstruction? Always assess the degree of upstream colonic distension and, in particular, try and detect any early signs of proximal mural compromise. Look for mural oedema and adjacent dirty fat around the caecal pole. Do not mistake air trapping for pneumatosis.
- Is there any evidence of complication, including perforation, abscess or fistula formation.
- Look for signs of portal pyaemia.
- If a pericolonic collection is present, is there a safe route for percutaneous drainage should this be the favoured clinical preference?

Recommended reading

Lawrimore T, Rhea JT. Computed tomography evaluation of diverticulitis. *J Intensive Care Med* 2004;19:194–204.

Lohrmann C, Ghanem N, Pache G, Makowiec F, Kotter E, Langer M. CT in acute perforated sigmoid diverticulitis. *Eur J Radiol* 2005;**56**:78–83.

Acute colitis

Summary

Protocol: Oral and IV contrast. Portal venous phase imaging.

What to look for: Colonic wall morphology and distribution of colonic involvement; any associated small bowel change; vascular tree abnormalities; complications such as obstruction or perforation, abscesses, fistulae to adjacent structures.

Report: Extent and severity of colitis, suggest likely aetiology, note any complications.

Acute colitis typically presents with abdominal pain and diarrhoea but may present more insidiously with vague abdominal discomfort and non-specific ill-health. Possible aetiologies include inflammatory bowel disease (ulcerative colitis and Crohn's disease), ischaemia, infection and immunocompromise. The CT findings often overlap and although a specific diagnosis can be offered in some circumstances, biopsy is often required to establish the final pathology.

Protocol and technique

Contrast enhancement:

- **Oral contrast:** Full abdominal and pelvic contrast generally using positive contrast. Rectal contrast is not part of the standard protocol, although it is preferred by some centres.
- **IV contrast:** 100 ml contrast delivered at 3 ml/s with images acquired in the portal venous phase.

Slice collimation: 2–5 mm axial reconstruction. Multiplanar reformatted images in the coronal plane can be helpful to illustrate the extent of the colitis and any associated complications.

What to look for on CT

- Establish the distribution of colonic disease, and look for any involvement of small bowel, particularly the terminal ileum.
- Establish the degree of colonic wall thickening and assess the mural density. Decide whether pathological thickening is minor or gross. Remember that colonic wall thickness depends on the degree of luminal distension, so do not overcall apparent thickening in a collapsed segment of colon. Placing undue reliance on specific measurements is largely unnecessary in the emergency setting. Eye ball assessment is usually sufficient to decide what is normal and what is abnormal, and an appreciation of mural density is helpful when trying to establish the likely aetiology of the colitis. This is best assessed by comparing the density of pathological bowel wall with sections of normal colon.
- Evaluate luminal distension, commenting on critical levels of distension and signs of obstruction.
- Identify complications and secondary involvement of adjacent structures. Look for ascites, abscess formation and any established fistula formation.
- Look for abnormal gas patterns; free gas within the peritoneum or retroperitoneum, intramural or portal venous gas. Use *wide windows* or the 'invert' function key to help identify extra-enteric gas. Beware of overcalling intramural gas in segments of bowel containing viscous semisolid content. Classically seen at the caecal pole, peripherally trapped intraluminal gas can mimic intramural change. This pitfall can usually be avoided by noting a lack of 'intramural' change anterior to the air–fluid interface. If doubt remains, turning the patient prone and performing a limited repeat series through the region of concern usually resolves the issue when the previously trapped air will typically change position.

Specific causes of acute colitis: CT findings

Inflammatory bowel disease

Crohn's disease and ulcerative colitis may be indistinguishable on radiological grounds, but the distribution pattern and certain CT signs can help differentiate the two subtypes. Approximately 5% of patients have an indeterminate inflammatory colitis with overlapping clinical, radiological and even pathological features.

- The colonic wall is typically thicker and denser in Crohn's colitis compared to ulcerative colitis, the latter being a more mucosal-based pathology (Figs 4.19, 4.20).
- Wall thickening in ulcerative colitis is typically continuous and symmetrical, whereas Crohn's disease displays asymmetrical and segmental involvement with characteristic 'skip' regions (Fig. 4.18). Although rectal sparing is typical for Crohn's disease, the finding of perianal inflammatory changes and perianal fistula formation would point strongly to a diagnosis of Crohn's.

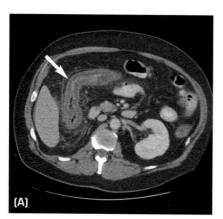
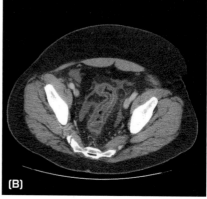

Figure 4.18: Ulcerative colitis. (A, B) Pancolitis showing low-density mural thickening with submucosal oedema, relatively minor perienteric inflammatory changes and only traces of ascites. **Differential diagnosis:** Pseudomembranous colitis could be considered here, and as always the history and clinical presentation is key to establishing a realistic differential diagnosis. In this case, note the prominent submucosal oedema (**A**, arrow), and the relatively well-preserved clarity to the outer mural margin when compared to the examples of pseudomembranous colitis. Always assess the terminal ileum – not illustrated here – when trying to differentiate between ulcerative colitis and Crohn's colitis. While backwash ileitis can lead to some confusion, the degree of mural thickening with Crohn's, along with enlarged loco-regional nodes and prominent vasa recta, should differentiate between the two conditions.

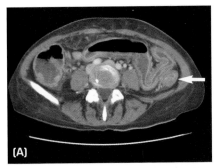

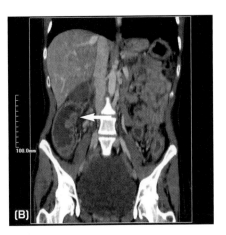

Figure 4.19: Ulcerative colitis. (A) Enhancing mucosa and submucosal oedema (arrow), typical of ulcerative colitis. **(B)** Inflammatory pseudopolyps in the ascending colon (arrow). Note again preservation of the outer mural margin clarity.

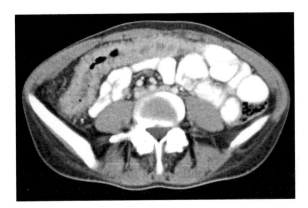

Figure 4.20: Crohn's colitis demonstrating higher density mural thickening when compared with ulcerative or infective colitis.

- Exclusive involvement of the right colon and small bowel is more commonly seen in Crohn's and infectious colitis than with ulcerative colitis. With pancolonic ulcerative colitis, terminal ileal involvement due to backwash ileitis may mimic Crohn's.
- In severe cases of ulcerative colitis, inflammatory pseudopolyps representing pronounced mucosal changes may be seen. These may be best appreciated on coronal reformats.
- Mesenteric fibrofatty proliferation is a feature of Crohn's disease, that can lead to local mass effect and separation of small bowel loops. *Submucosal* fat deposition is more frequently seen in ulcerative colitis. This produces the 'halo' sign, a low attenuation ring in the bowel wall due to deposition of low-density fat in the submucosa.

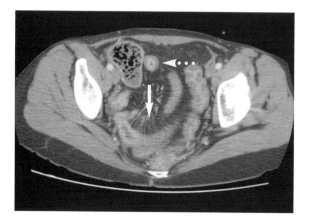

Figure 4.21: Crohn's disease. Terminal ileal mural thickening (dotted arrow) with small bowel involvement extending into the distal ileal loops. Note prominent vasa recta (arrow) in a patient with acute Crohn's colitis.

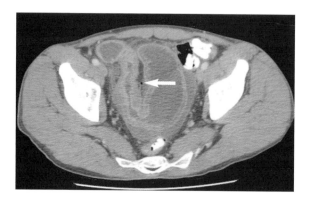

Figure 4.22: Crohn's disease complicated by perforation. Distal small bowel Crohn's with dilatation of the proximal loops and a fleck of extraluminal gas (arrow) lying between two involved loops of small bowel.

- Three other signs are more commonly found with Crohn's colitis and should be carefully looked for: prominence of the vasa recta (comb-like arrangement of the engorged vascular arcades in the small bowel mesentery), enhancing locoregional lymph nodes and perienteric abscess formation (Fig. 4.21).
- Uncommonly, bowel perforation may be the presenting feature of inflammatory bowel disease (Fig. 4.22). Always consider this diagnosis when a young patient presents with free intraperitoneal gas and an inflammatory mass in the right iliac fossa. Nevertheless, a perforated appendiceal mass would remain the more probable diagnosis, the final pathology only being established at surgery. Other complications can occur in Crohn's disease (Fig. 4.23).
- Look for critical levels of colonic distension. Toxic megacolon (sometimes known as acute toxic colitis), representing non-obstructed distension of the colon, is an emergency and requires urgent discussion with the referring clinician. The caecum is the most distensible section of colon (see later under large bowel obstruction) and most

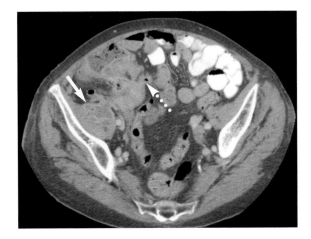

**Figure 4.23:
Complicated Crohn's
disease.** Fistulous
tracts extending into
the mesentery
medially (dotted arrow)
and the right iliacus
muscle laterally with
focal abscess
formation (arrow).

prevelant to perforation when toxic dilatation develops. Caecal diameters of 9 cm plus are worrisome, with diameters of 12–14 cm representing critical levels of distension. Colonic distension, along with signs of systemic illness, should suggest this diagnosis, which can be a life-threatening complication found with any of the colitides.

- Ascites is not a prominent finding in inflammatory bowel disease.
- Look for other pathology associated with inflammatory bowel disease, such as sacroileitis and sclerosing cholangitis. These findings are usually seen with chronic established disease.

Pseudomembranous (infective) colitis (Fig. 4.24)

Infective colitis (commonly caused by *Clostridium difficile*) is currently responsible for an increasing hospital morbidity and mortality, particularly in the elderly. The reported sensitivity of CT for the diagnosis of *C. difficile* colitis is around 50%. Serological titres may be negative in approximately one-third, and the typical pseudomembranes may be absent on initial sigmoidoscopy. Not infrequently, the condition is unsuspected by the referring clinician and the radiologist may be the first to suggest the diagnosis when classical CT signs are present:

- Prominent colonic wall thickening is a characteristic finding with mural thickness often in excess of 10 mm. Mural density is typically low, reflecting the presence of extensive oedema, but high-density changes may also be observed. The 'accordion' sign describes oral contrast trapped between thickened colonic folds. This sign is not specific for infective colitis and may be found in other forms of severe colitis.
- Disease distribution may be pancolonic or limited to the left colon, right colon, caecum or rectum in order of decreasing frequency. *C. difficile* enteritis is exceedingly rare, but with the current increasing

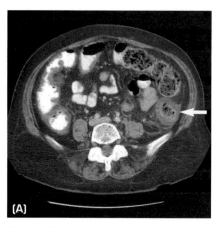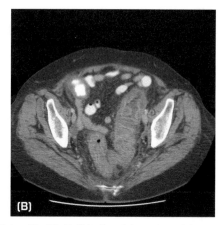

(A) (B)

Figure 4.24: Pseudomembranous colitis. (A, B) Colitis involving sigmoid, descending and ascending colon with sparing of distal transverse colon and splenic flexure. Features supporting a diagnosis of pseudomembranous colitis are (1) the degree of mural thickening, i.e. at the more prominent end of the colitis spectrum, and (2) the low density of the mural changes, best shown in the descending colon (arrow) and sigmoid.

prevalence of infectious colitis in our hospital populations, this diagnosis should be considered when distal small bowel changes are noted in addition to colitic changes in the appropriate clinical setting.
- Free intraperitoneal fluid is an expected finding along with prominent pericolonic inflammatory stranding.
- Acute toxic colitis can also complicate infectious colitis.

Neutropenic colitis (Fig. 4.25)

Neutropenic sepsis should always be considered in the differential of colitis when there is any likelihood of immunocompromise. A supporting history is fundamental to this diagnosis as the CT features are rather non-specific.

- Marked mural thickening with superficial ulcerations usually confined to the caecum and ascending colon, along with pericolonic fat stranding of varying severity.
- Abscess formation, haemorrhage, intestinal necrosis and frank perforation may occur in severe cases.

Ischaemic colitis

Atrial fibrillation, cardiac dysfunction, generalized arteriopathy and post-prandial abdominal pain should alert the radiologist to the possibility of intestinal ischaemia being the cause of the colitis. Ischaemia,

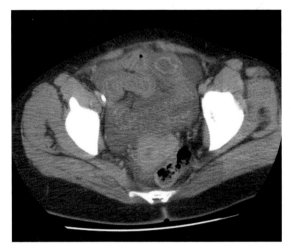

Figure 4.25:
Neutropaenic colitis.
Patient admitted with sepsis and a low white cell count. Pancolitis with mainly low-density mural thickening (in this example best illustrated in the sigmoid colon) and prominent ascites. Neutropaenic colitis was confirmed following colonoscopy and biopsy. Infectious colitis could give comparable appearances.

whether secondary to thrombotic or embolic events, typically affects the so-called watershed territories (areas of deficient collateral blood supply), such as the distal transverse colon and distal descending colon. The rectosigmoid junction and splenic flexure are particularly vulnerable. Ischaemic colitis is usually arterial in origin, but can be secondary to venous compromise.

Although CT is the imaging method of choice for assessing acute intestinal ischaemia, the diagnosis can be difficult to make in the early stages when the CT signs can be rather non-specific. Early venous infarction is a particularly difficult call. Ischaemia may not have been considered by the referring clinician and it may be down to the radiologist to suggest the diagnosis.

- Look for segmental or diffuse bowel wall thickening, 'thumb printing' (indentations on the bowel wall contour resembling thumb marks) and pericolonic stranding in the watershed areas.
- The degree of mural thickening with ischaemic bowel can be variable and is typically more pronounced with venous than with arterial occlusion. With total vascular occlusion and no reperfusion (i.e. infarction), the colonic wall is usually thin with reduced or absent contrast enhancement. There may be associated luminal dilatation and occasionally a toxic megacolon picture develops.
- Mural density is similarly variable and can range from essentially normal, to high (representing intramural haemorrhage), to low (representing submucosal oedema).
- Carefully follow the mesenteric arterial and venous channels looking for thrombus or occlusion, to confirm the diagnosis. Try to follow the vascular branches to each quadrant of the abdomen but be careful not to assume occlusive change in severely arteriopathic patients is

Summary of key diagnostic features in colitis

Assess the extent and distribution of the colitis, the wall thickness, the wall density and the mural enhancement pattern.

Wall thickening:
- Accept that the assessment of wall thickness can be difficult and largely subjective in the absence of colonic cleansing or adequate distension.
- Suggest 'major' or 'minor' mural thickening rather than reporting specific mural measurements.
- With major wall thickening, consider pseudomembranous, Crohn's or neutropenic colitis as possible diagnoses.
- With minor wall thickening, consider ulcerative colitis and radiation colitis.
- Unfortunately, ischaemia can produce the whole spectrum of mural thickening and density changes found with other colitides.

Mural density in colitis:
- Low attenuation: pseudomembranous (infective) colitis
- High attenuation: consider Crohn's and ischaemic colitis while accepting the variations found with ischaemia.
- 'Target' appearance, reflecting the submucosal oedema found with ulcerative colitis.

Submucosal oedema:
- Prominent finding in ulcerative colitis.
- Less prominent in pseudomembranous and Crohn's colitis.
- Not usually recognized in ischaemic and radiation colitis.

Ascites:
- Frequent finding with infectious colitis.
- Less often seen in inflammatory bowel disease and radiation colitis, and may be absent in early ischaemic colitis.

Pneumatosis:
- Usually associated with bowel ischaemia, but may occasionally be seen in severe ulcerative colitis.

always acute. Consider the possibility that atheromatous occlusion or partial compromise may reflect chronic rather than acute disease.
- Ischaemic bowel can appear flaccid and atonic with stagnant-appearing intraluminal content.
- Ascites is usually present.
- 'Pneumatosis coli' and/or portal venous gas are secondary effects of bowel infarction. Pneumatosis is seen as punctuate or linear foci of air

in the intestinal wall and is best appreciated on a wide window or by using the invert function key on the workstation. Look specifically for non-dependent mural gas. Carefully review the mesenteric veins for any venous gas and trace to the superior mesenteric, splenic and portal veins, then into the liver. Look for the characteristic 'bird's claw' peripheral branching gas pattern within the liver.

Radiation colitis

A history of radiation exposure is crucial here as CT findings may be non-specific. Acute radiation injury to the colon occurs within a few weeks of exposure and usually presents as self-limiting diarrhoea.

- CT changes are often similar to colonic ischaemia but localized to anatomy covered by the radiation port.
- Mural density can be heterogenous rather than uniform.
- Rectal wall thickening and perienteric oedema develop in the acute stages with increased intramural and perirectal fat seen in the chronic phase.
- Stricturing and fistula formation are recognized long-term complications.
- There may be similar changes affecting adjacent small bowel loops if exposed by the same radiation port.

Differential diagnosis

Any acute intra-abdominal inflammatory pathology may lead to secondary colonic changes that can mimic a primary colitis. Focal or localized colonic thickening may be found with acute cholecystitis and appendicitis, whereas in acute pancreatitis, the bowel changes may be focal or more extensive.

Acute reporting

- Describe the extent and severity of the colitis.
- Suggest the likely aetiology based on the history and your findings.
- Identify and report complications such as toxic dilatation, obstruction, perforation, abscess formation and fistula formation.

Recommended reading
Thoeni RF, Cello JP. CT imaging of colitis. *Radiology* 2006;240:623–38.

Small bowel obstruction

Summary

Protocol: No oral contrast necessary. IV contrast with imaging in portal venous phase.

What to look for: Dilated fluid-filled proximal small bowel, collapsed distal small bowel and the point of transition. Look for signs of closed loop obstruction or vascular compromise.

Report: Site and cause of obstruction and any complications.

Intestinal obstruction accounts for about 20% of all admissions for acute abdominal pain with about 80% involving the small bowel. Common causes of obstruction include postoperative adhesions (~60%), external or internal hernias (~15%), neoplasms (~15%) and other causes (~10%), including inflammatory bowel disease, trauma, intussusception, gallstones, foreign bodies and endometriosis. CT has a sensitivity of 94% and specificity of 96% for the detection of small bowel obstruction.

Protocol and technique

Contrast enhancement:

- **Oral contrast:** Not usually required as fluid in obstructed small bowel provides natural contrast for diagnosis. Insisting that oral contrast is given to a vomiting obstructed patient is not recommended.
- **IV contrast:** Images are acquired during the portal venous phase of contrast enhancement. 100 ml contrast at 3 ml/s.

Slice collimation: 2.5–5 mm axial reconstructions. Coronal and sagittal reformats as required. Coverage from diaphragm down to the perineum. Ensure the hernial orifices and obturator canals are included.

What to look for on CT

- Confirm small bowel obstruction; look for the diagnostic combination of dilated fluid-filled proximal small bowel and collapsed distal small bowel.
- Identify the transition zone which lies at the junction between those dilated and air/fluid-filled loops proximal to the site of obstruction and the collapsed loops distal to the obstruction. Multiplanar reformatted images can help identify this point.

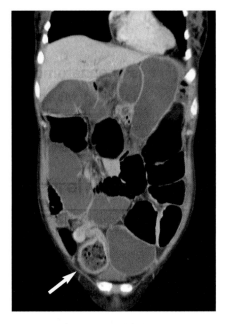

Figure 4.26: Small bowel obstruction secondary to post-surgical adhesions. Classical proximal fluid-filled dilated small bowel and collapsed distal loops. Note the small bowel faeces sign just proximal to the transition zone (arrow).

■ The 'small bowel faeces' sign is another aid to finding the transition point. This describes the presence of particulate faeculent matter mixed with gas bubbles in that section of small bowel immediately proximal to the point of obstruction and is due to delayed intestinal transit causing digestion of food and bacterial overgrowth (Fig. 4.26).

■ Try and establish a likely aetiology for the obstruction such as a hernia, enterolith, or gallstone. The commoner causes of small bowel obstruction are listed below (see box and Figs 4.27, 4.28, 4.29).

■ When no obvious cause is found, and there is a history of previous abdominal or pelvic surgery, adhesions will be the likely diagnosis. If a virgin abdomen and no apparent cause, consider a congenital band.

■ Gas in the biliary tree along with signs of small bowel obstruction should always suggest a diagnosis of gallstone ileus. Two caveats need consideration; first there are other potential reasons for biliary tree gas and second, biliary tree gas does not always accompany gallstone ileus. It will in the majority, but its absence should not mean the diagnosis is excluded. Clinical correlation is essential (Figs 4.30, 4.31).

■ When gas is identified in the biliary tree, look for supporting evidence of a fistula between the biliary tree or gallbladder and adjacent small bowel. Look carefully for the obstructing gallstone which will usually be found at the point of small bowel obstruction. Multiplanar reformats can be helpful here.

■ Discriminate between biliary tree gas and portal venous gas. The former tends to be more central, contrasting with the more peripheral

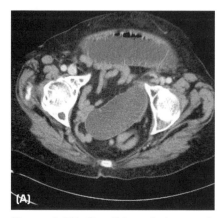
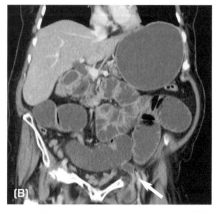

Figure 4.27: Small bowel obstruction secondary to an inguinal hernia. (A) Note both dilated and collapsed small bowel loops on the axial image. (B) Coronal reformats demonstrate the site and cause of obstruction (arrow). Note the excellent natural contrast provided by the small bowel fluid, illustrating why oral contrast is not required.

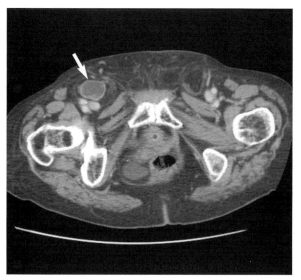

Figure 4.28: Right femoral hernia (arrow) as the cause of small bowel obstruction. Always ensure dilated small bowel can be shown to enter the hernia with collapsed small bowel exiting the hernia. Never assume an incidental asymptomatic hernia with an absence of the above features is the cause of the patient's acute presentation.

subcapsular location of portal vein gas. Thin, branching, gas-filled structures extending to within a centimetre or less of the capsular surface are typical findings for portal vein gas.

- What is the severity of obstruction? Decide whether high- or low-grade obstruction is present. This can be a subjective call but the presence of a clear abrupt transition between significantly dilated and collapsed small bowel indicates a likely need for surgical inter-

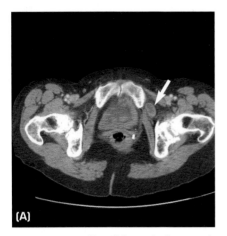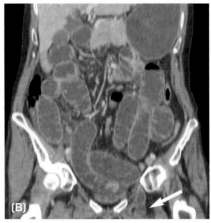

Figure 4.29: Small bowel obstruction caused by obturator hernia
(arrows). (A, B) Classical appearance and location. Always ensure the
hernial orifices are covered on the scanning protocol.

vention. Ascites typically accompanies high-grade obstruction and
always look for signs of ischaemia. Subacute small bowel obstruction
is usually associated with more modest degrees of small bowel dilatation and in this situation, some radiologists find giving oral contrast
helpful. The passage of contrast into the right colon confirms incomplete obstruction with conservative management remaining an
option.

■ Is there a closed loop obstruction? By definition, a closed loop obstruction indicates occlusion at two adjacent points along a segment of
small bowel and is usually secondary to adhesions or an internal hernia. Look for a dilated loop of small bowel with a 'U'-shaped or kidney
bean configuration. A 'beak sign' may be identified, which represents
tapering of the obstructed loop at the point of compromise.

■ When small bowel volvulus develops, the bowel loops adopt a radial
configuration accompanied by engorged mesenteric vessels and associated mesenteric oedema converging towards the point of obstruction
in a characteristic whirl pattern. Be careful not to overcall the whirl
pattern. Normal mesenteric vessels can produce whirling configurations in the absence of pathology. Significant whirling is usually
accompanied by vascular engorgement and oedema.

■ Are there any features of strangulation? Strangulation means
ischaemic compromise has developed, and is often accompanied by a
closed loop situation. Look for localised, wedge shaped areas of
oedema in the mesentery subtending the obstructed section of small
bowel. When found, this strongly suggests ischaemic compromise.
Look for pneumatosis and in the later stages, free intraperitoneal gas

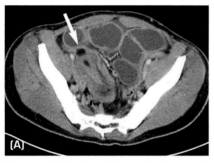

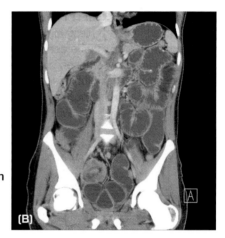

Figure 4.30: Small bowel obstruction caused by intussusception. (A, B) A lipoma (arrow) was thought to be the lead point.

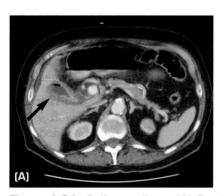

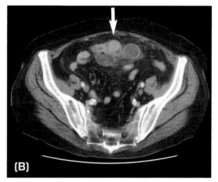

Figure 4.31: Gallstone ileus. (A) Gas in the gallbladder (arrow) and pericholecystic fluid. **(B)** An impacted gallstone in the small bowel just proximal to the transition zone between the dilated and collapsed small bowel (arrow).

and portal venous gas. Refer to the section on bowel ischaemia above for further detail.

Differential diagnosis

Small bowel ileus is the main differential from mechanical small bowel obstruction. With ileus, there is global dilatation throughout the small bowel without a transition zone. Ileus usually develops after abdominal surgery or when there is a background of physiological or biochemical dysfunction. In the majority of cases, dilatation of the ascending and transverse colon will also be noted (see section above on large bowel obstruction).

Causes of small bowel obstruction

Extrinsic causes:
- Adhesions
- Hernia
- Appendicitis
- Diverticulitis
- Carcinoid
- Lymphoma
- Peritoneal carcinomatosis

Intrinsic causes:
- Crohn's disease
- Adenocarcinoma
- Intussusception
- Tuberculosis
- Radiation enteropathy
- Intramural haemorrhage

Intraluminal causes:
- Gallstones
- Bezoars
- Foreign body
- Round worm

Intestinal malrotation

Acute reporting

- Determine if small bowel obstruction is present or not.
- Identify the level: suggest proximal, mid or distal small bowel when the transition point is difficult to find. Remember location is not an absolute guide to small bowel anatomy. Jejunal loops may lie in the pelvis and ileal loops towards the left upper quadrant.
- Give an indication of severity: High-grade, subacute, closed loop, strangulation.
- Look for complications such as perforation.
- Suggest an aetiology if there are CT findings that indicate a specific diagnosis.

Recommended reading

Furukawa A, Yamasaki M, Furuichi K, et al. Helical CT in the diagnosis of small bowel obstruction. *Radiographics* 2001;**21**:341–55.

Mallo RD, Salem L, Lalani T, Flum DR. Computed tomography diagnosis of ischemia and complete obstruction in small bowel obstruction: a systematic review. *J Gastrointest Surg* 2005;**9**:690–4.

Qalbani A, Paushter D, Dachman AH. Multidetector row CT of small bowel obstruction. *Radiol Clin North Am* 2007;45:499–512, viii.

Large bowel obstruction

Summary

Protocol: No oral contrast required. IV contrast with imaging in portal venous phase.

What to look for: Confirm level and look for cause of obstruction. Differentiate from pseudo-obstruction. Are there signs of ischaemic compromise and/or perforation? If malignancy is detected, identify any extra-colonic spread.

Report: Include the above information. Discuss any need for urgent intervention or need for water-soluble enema if doubt remains as to whether true obstruction or pseudo-obstruction.

Mechanical large bowel obstruction is a clinical emergency requiring early detection and intervention. Large bowel obstruction may be of gradual onset, such as secondary to an obstructing neoplasm or complicated diverticulitis, or of more abrupt onset when due to an acute volvulus. The early diagnosis of large bowel obstruction is critical to prevent complications such as perforation and ischaemia. CT will detect the location and often the cause of obstruction, as well as identifying complications. CT has largely replaced the traditional role of water-soluble enema and is particularly useful and much kinder in the frail, unwell and elderly patients who would have difficulty tolerating an enema.

Pseudo-obstruction is a condition of differing aetiology and management options that must be distinguished from true obstruction using clinical and imaging criteria. Pseudo-obstruction, sometimes known as Ogilvie syndrome or acute colonic ileus, typically occurs in debilitated patients with medical or surgical problems, and the mean prevalence is in the seventh and eighth decades. It is defined as a condition with the symptoms, signs and radiological appearances of large bowel obstruction without a demonstrable mechanical cause. Abdominal distension is the major clinical finding.

Protocol and technique

Contrast enhancement:

- **Oral contrast:** Not required as fluid and gas in obstructed bowel provide sufficient natural contrast.
- **IV contrast**: 100 ml at 3 ml/s. Images are acquired in the portal venous phase of contrast enhancement.

Slice collimation: 2.5–5 mm axial images. Coverage from diaphragm to symphysis pubis.

What to look for on CT

- Confirm obstruction. Large bowel calibre is variable and there are no universally accepted criteria for pathological dilatation. As a guide, a colonic diameter of > 6 cm (9 cm in the caecum as it is more distensible) is generally considered significant. As with small bowel obstruction, identifying the point of calibre change between dilated and collapsed bowel is the key observation. If the ileocaecal valve is incompetent, dilated small bowel loops may accompany large bowel obstruction.
- Locate the transition point (Fig. 4.32). Follow the colon retrogradely from the rectum to the caecum, looking for an abrupt change in calibre. Alternatively locate the ileocaecal valve and follow the colon from the ascending colon to the rectum. Multiplanar reformats, particularly in the coronal plane can be helpful. On occasion, following convoluted loops of sigmoid may be difficult and tracing the colon from

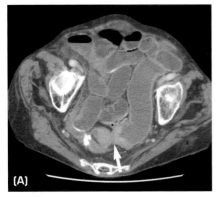 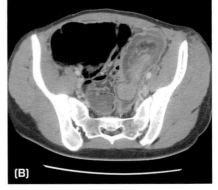

Figure 4.32: Large bowel obstruction. (A) Bowel obstruction secondary to a distal sigmoid colonic carcinoma (arrow). **(B)** Large bowel obstruction caused by a colocolonic intussusception secondary to a colonic polyp.

both ends may be necessary to clarify the anatomy. In the pelvis, always establish which are colonic loops and which are small bowel loops before reaching a firm diagnosis. As with the interpretation of small bowel anatomy, sorting out the colonic road map is a much simpler exercise on the diagnostic console or PACS monitor than reviewing on hard copy.

■ Comment on the severity of obstruction and complications if any. Perforation and intestinal ischaemia are the major causes of morbidity and mortality in patients with large bowel obstruction. Ischaemia is mainly a result of venous compromise secondary to increased intraluminal pressure. Look for mural thickening and gas in the bowel wall. At an earlier stage, more subtle findings may be present, especially involving the distended caecal pole when pericolonic oedema and reduced mural clarity may be noted. This finding must alert the radiologist to the possibility of early serosal compromise, leading to tears and perforation if the obstruction is not swiftly relieved.

■ Frank perforation will result in **faecal peritonitis**. The caecum is the most common site of large bowel perforation. LaPlace's law states that the pressure required to stretch the walls of a hollow viscus decreases in inverse proportion to the radius of curvature of the viscus. Therefore, as the caecum will have the largest diameter, it will be the first site to succumb to increasing pressure. When caecal diameters reach 12–14 cm, the risk of perforation becomes critical.

■ Try and suggest the likely aetiology. The commonest causes are colonic carcinoma and diverticular disease, with sigmoid and caecal volvulus, ischaemia and inflammatory bowel disease also to be considered. Less common causes include hernias, intussusception and bezoars.

■ *Volvulus:* Volvulus is the third leading cause of mechanical large bowel obstruction and results from twisting an intestinal loop around itself. The large bowel is particularly vulnerable to volvulus due to the narrow attachment of its mesentery to the posterior abdominal wall. When volvulus develops, the two adjacent limbs of the compromised large bowel are seen on CT as a dilated 'U'-shaped distended viscus which narrows at the point of twisting. Confirming that the caecum lies in its normal anatomical position will help differentiate a caecal from a sigmoid volvulus. Multiplanar images can also help when trying to discriminate between the two types of volvulus.

Differential diagnosis

■ *Pseudo-obstruction:* Pseudo-obstruction represents benign colonic dilatation not associated with a mechanical cause. With pseudo-obstruction, the right hemicolon and transverse colon are dilated, a colonic calibre change occurs just distal to the splenic flexure, and the remainder of the colon is generally collapsed. The site of calibre change can be more distal involving the lower descending colon or even sigmoid. Occasionally, it can be impossible to confidently eliminate a true stricture at the point of luminal change and if so, a limited water-soluble contrast enema will be needed to exclude mechanical obstruction. The contrast only needs to be run to a point proximal to the area of concern as the rest of the colon has been cleared by CT.

■ **Generalized ileus:** Generalized ileus typically shows as pan small bowel dilatation with colonic dilatation to splenic flexure and collapsed colon thereafter. Distinguishing generalized ileus and colonic ileus is not important. The important differentiation is between true obstruction and pseudo-obstruction of the large bowel.

Interventional aspects

Acute colonic stent placement may be used as an alternative to surgery to relieve large bowel obstruction in patients where immediate acute surgery is considered inadvisable or inappropriate. Colonic stenting is indicated for primary and recurrent colonic malignancy or extrinsic malignancy leading to colonic stricturing. Stents are typically deployed for left colon pathology with access difficulties limiting right colon placement. Currently, stenting is not indicated for benign disease and is not appropriate for lower or middle third rectal tumours.

Acute reporting

■ Confirm or exclude the diagnosis of large bowel obstruction.
■ Document the site and if possible, the cause of the obstruction.
■ Note any complications such as perforation.
■ If due to an obvious malignancy, give an indication of the extent of any extracolonic and distant spread.
■ If you cannot confidently differentiate between obstruction and pseudo-obstruction, discuss the option of a limited water-soluble contrast enema with the referring clinician.

Recommended reading

Khurana B, Ledbetter S, McTavish J, Wiesner W, Ros PR. Bowel obstruction revealed by multidetector CT. *AJR Am J Roentgenol* 2002;**178**: 1139–44.

Sinha R, Verma R. Multidetector row computed tomography in bowel obstruction. Part 2. Large bowel obstruction. *Clin Radiol* 2005;**60**:1068–75.

Acute bowel ischaemia

Summary

Protocol: Oral and IV contrast. Image in portal venous phase.

What to look for: Abnormal bowel wall thickening and density, mesenteric vascular occlusion, pneumatosis/portal venous gas/intraperitoneal gas.

Report: Location and extent of bowel ischaemia.

Acute mesenteric ischaemia can be a difficult diagnosis to make on both clinical and radiological criteria. Ischaemia develops when enteric blood flow (arterial or venous) is critically compromised. About 1% of all patients presenting with an acute abdomen will have bowel ischaemia as the cause. MDCT is ideally suited to provide a comprehensive assessment of the bowel anatomy and the mesenteric vasculature using thin section axial and multiplanar images. The sensitivity and specificity of MDCT for the detection of acute mesenteric ischaemia is reported to be as high as 92% and 100%, respectively. Nevertheless, although diagnosis is straightforward when the classical findings are present, but in the early stages of ischaemia, especially with venous infarction, interpretation can be more difficult.

Protocol and technique

Contrast enhancement:

- **Oral contrast:** It is down to local preference whether oral contrast is given. In the majority of cases, the diagnosis of ischaemia will be sug-

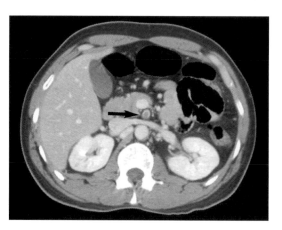

Figure 4.33: Bowel ischaemia. Acute superior mesenteric artery thrombosis. Note the filling defect in the superior mesenteric artery (arrow).

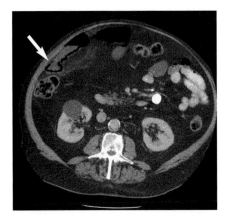

Figure 4.34: Small bowel ischaemia. Note the intramural air (arrow) in a loop of small bowel showing no recognizable wall enhancement. The wedge-shaped configuration of the adjacent mesenteric oedema is a typical finding with small bowel ischaemia.

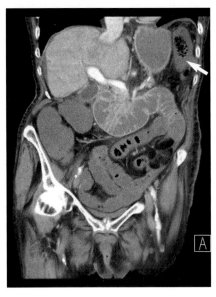

Figure 4.35: Acute ischaemia large and small bowel. Patient who presented with sudden onset abdominal pain. Coronal image shows mural enhancement of only the proximal jejunal loops, contrasting with the more distal small bowel loops that show no mural enhancement. Unusually in this example, perienteric oedema and ascites is minimal. Other sections showed limited mural gas. Note the mural thickening and non-enhancement to the splenic flexure (arrow), indicating further ischaemic compromise. Other sections confirmed global colonic ischaemia.

gested during a survey study of the abdomen when no firm clinical decision has been made, and oral contrast will form part of the standard acute protocol. When ischaemia is thought the most likely clinical diagnosis, either positive or negative contrast can be used, although negative contrast has definite advantages when it comes to assessing bowel wall morphology and enhancement characteristics.

- **Intravenous contrast:** Imaging in portal venous phase. 100 ml at 3 ml/s. Dual arterial and portal venous phase imaging does not offer any significant advantage.

Slice collimation: 2.5–5 mm reconstructed axial sections. Multiplanar reformatted images using the thinner section source data can be very helpful for diagnosis.

What to look for on CT (Figs 4.33–4.35)

- Evaluate the bowel wall and look for mural thickening and density changes. Bowel wall density may be reduced due to submucosal oedema or increased due to submucosal haemorrhage. Both are recognized findings but remember in the early stages of ischaemia the bowel wall may appear fairly normal. Circumferential thickening is one of the commonest CT features of an ischaemic segment. The thickened bowel wall may have a 'target sign' appearance, i.e. alternating layers of high and low attenuation corresponding to submucosal haemorrhage and oedema respectively.

- Review the mesenteric arterial and venous vascular arcades and look for focal filling defects or vascular occlusion. It can be difficult to decide which changes are acute and which are chronic when extensive background arteriopathy is present. Follow the mesenteric vascular tree from the central major vessels to the distal branches of each abdominal quadrant. This is best achieved on the diagnostic workstation and again coronal reformats are particularly helpful when following the vascular arcades.

- In patients with atrial fibrillation, short segment involvement or multifocal bowel involvement may be recognized, reflecting the effect of embolic showers (Fig. 4.37). Review the axial sections through the lower chest – you might recognize a metallic heart valve.

- Ascites is a common finding, but its absence does not exclude the possibility of ischaemia.

- Localized mesenteric oedema is a very important sign and usually accompanies localized change in bowel wall morphology. Look for characteristic often triangular, wedge-like areas of mesenteric oedema subtending a segment of abnormal bowel. The presence of localized mesenteric oedema in a triangular distribution should trigger consideration of ischaemia as the primary diagnosis.

- Pneumatosis is a late feature of ischaemia and more often than not indicates irreversibility of the process. Gas within mesenteric and intrahepatic portal vein branches are secondary features. Remember intrahepatic portal vein gas tends to extend close to the liver capsule in a dependent peripheral distribution. Biliary gas tends to be more prominent centrally and can usually be recognized within the extrahepatic biliary tree. Only rarely does differentiating between the two entities become a problem.

- Identify flaccid and atonic appearing segments of small bowel that might also show intraluminal gas concentrated within a more central position rather than in the more expected dependent distribution. These are features of aperistaltic bowel with stagnant content, and when accompanied by wall morphology showing reduced or absent enhancement, are strong indicators of likely ischaemia.

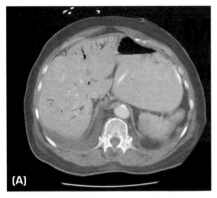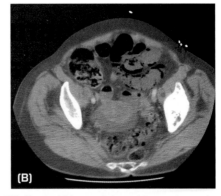

(A) (B)

Figure 4.36: Small bowel ischaemia. (A) Gas within peripheral branches of the intrahepatic portal vein (note the gas is extending close to the periphery of liver while the biliary gas is characteristically located in more central position). **(B)** Mural gas within a pelvic small bowel loop.

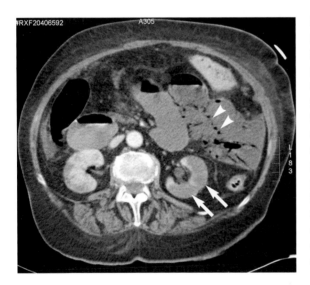

Figure 4.37: Embolic small bowel infarction. Elderly patient who presented with abdominal pain and new-onset atrial fibrillation. Multiple non-enhancing left-sided small bowel loops with non-dependent mural gas (arrowheads). Both kidneys show areas of reduced cortical enhancement consistent with areas of infarction.

- Thinning of the bowel wall and subsequent perforation are late findings and often herald the onset of peritoneal sepsis.
- When ischaemia develops secondary to small bowel obstruction, i.e. strangulated obstruction, identify the level of obstruction and suggest a likely aetiology.

Differential diagnosis

As mentioned earlier, the imaging findings of bowel ischemia can be non-specific, especially in the early stages, and bowel wall thickening is

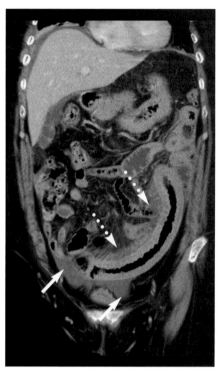

Figure 4.38: Small bowel mural haemorrhage. Patient presented with a 4-day history of abdominal pain. Current medication included warfarin for a recent deep vein thrombosis. Clotting status on admission was grossly deranged. Coronal CT image shows a 25-cm segment of high-density small bowel mural thickening. Note high-density fluid in the mesentery adjacent to the abnormal loop (dotted arrows). Also, note high-density ascites (arrows) reflecting haemoperitoneum. Small bowel ischaemia was considered in the differential diagnosis but the high-density changes within the bowel mesentery are atypical. Histological examination of the resected segment confirmed intramural haemorrhage with no coexisting pathology, leaving a diagnosis of spontaneous small bowel haemorrhage secondary to uncontrolled anticoagulation. This is a rare but well recognized complication of warfarin therapy.

recognized in a number of acute abdominal conditions. Any suggested differential requires careful correlation with other imaging findings as well as the presenting and past medical history. Consider:

- Inflammatory bowel disease.
- Infectious enteropathy, particularly if immunocompromised.
- Small bowel haemorrhage (Fig. 4.38).
- Radiation enteropathy.

Interventional aspects

Close liaison with the vascular radiologists is required as early thrombolytic therapy is reported to be an effective technique for potentially salvageable bowel ischaemia that is accompanied by definite CT evidence of vascular occlusion. However, in the majority of centres, conventional surgery remains the preferred mode of management.

Acute reporting

- Describe the location, extent and severity of bowel involvement.
- Comment on associated features such as ascites, pneumatosis and mesenteric or portal venous gas.
- Is there a definite cause, such as vascular occlusion or strangulated obstruction?
- The final decision to operate will always lie with the surgeon. In general terms, it is preferable for the radiologist to overcall rather than undercall any concerns of ischaemia. A delayed radiological diagnosis is generally a diagnosis too late for the patient.

Recommended reading

Cademartiri F, Raaijmakers RH, Kuiper JW, van Dijk LC, Pattynama PM, Krestin GP. Multi-detector row CT angiography in patients with abdominal angina. *Radiographics* 2004;**24**:969–84.

Horton KM, Fishman EK. Multi-detector row CT of mesenteric ischemia: Can it be done? *Radiographics* 2001;**21**:1463–73.

Renal colic

Summary

Protocol: Unenhanced study covering kidneys, ureters and bladder.

What to look for: Renal, ureteric, bladder calculi. Signs of renal tract compromise, i.e. peri-renal and peri-ureteric oedema, hydronephrosis. If the renal tracts appear normal, look for other causes of acute abdominal pain.

Report: Location and size of calculi. Note associated complications, such as hydronephrosis and hydroureter. Indicate alternative diagnostic options for abdominal pain.

Renal colic is a common cause of acute abdominal pain. Unenhanced CT of the urinary system (CT KUB) is highly sensitive and specific (over 96%) for the detection of renal and ureteric calculi, and has become the standard investigation for suspected acute renal colic. Ultrasound remains the preferred first option in the young female population and the acute intravenous urogram is now largely a historical investigation.

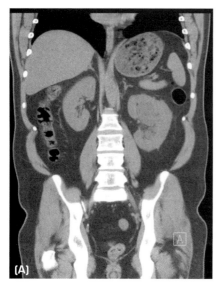 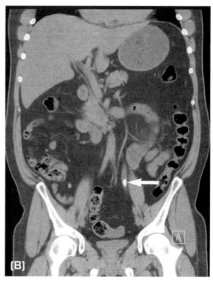

Figure 4.39: Renal colic. (A, B) The left kidney is hydronephrotic with an obstructing calculus in the ipsilateral mid-ureter (arrow). The coronal display is helpful to the clinician for planning management.

Protocol and technique

Ensure that the urinary bladder is full. Scanning in the **prone position** helps differentiate between a calculus impacted at the vesicoureteric junction and one free within the bladder.

Contrast enhancement: No oral or IV contrast is generally required. IV contrast is not part of the standard acute stone chasing protocol but occasionally may be used at times of diagnostic uncertainty. Acute renal or perirenal changes with no renal tract calcification might suggest either the presence of a non-radio-opaque calculus or alternatively, acute pyelonephritis as the cause of the abdominal pain.

Slice collimation: 2.5–5 mm reconstructed axial sections covering the kidneys, ureters and bladder. Coronal reformatted images using the source dataset can provide a useful road map for urological planning.

What to look for on CT

- Look for **high-attenuation calculi** in the kidneys, ureters or bladder. The majority of renal tract calculi are radio-opaque (Figs 4.39–4.41).
- The maximum axial measurement of a calculus should be recorded. This will give an indication as to whether a calculus should pass spontaneously (<5 mm) or might require intervention (>5 mm).

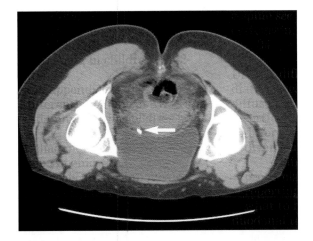

Figure 4.40: Renal colic. Prone image showing 5 mm calculus (arrow) at the vesicoureteric junction in a patient presenting with right-sided renal colic. Prone imaging is helpful when trying to establish whether a stone remains within the distal ureter or lies free within the bladder lumen.

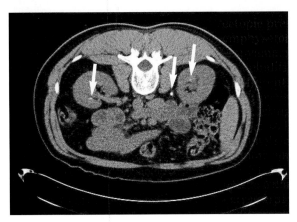

Figure 4.41: Renal colic. Unenhanced CT image illustrating the advantages of CT in diagnosing low-volume calculi that are unlikely to be identified on conventional abdominal radiographs. Tiny calculi in both kidneys and upper left ureter (arrows).

- Differentiating between a true ureteric calculus and an adjacent pelvic phlebolith can be difficult, especially when there is a lack of intrapelvic fat. The 'tissue rim' sign can help. Look for a rim of soft tissue attenuation representing the oedematous ureteric wall surrounding a calcific density. This sign usually develops within 4–24 h of obstruction and is useful for differentiating small stones from phleboliths. Pelvic side wall vascular calcification can also be a source of diagnostic doubt.
- When doubt remains as to whether a calculus lies within the ureter or not (Figs 4.40, 4.41), or if there is the suspicion that a stone might have already passed, look for the secondary signs:
  - ☐ Perinephric or periureteric stranding.
  - ☐ Renal enlargement and blurring of the renal outline.
  - ☐ Hydronephrosis and/or hydroureter.
  - ☐ Urinoma formation, indicating rupture of an obstructed system (Fig. 4.42).

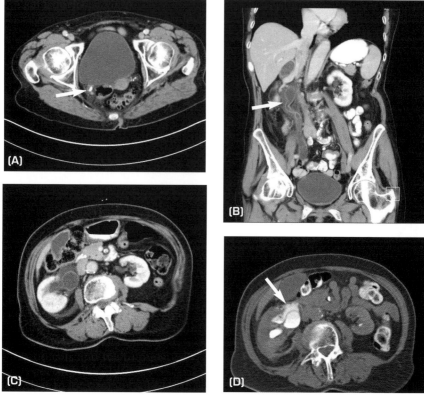

Figure 4.42: Complicated urolithiasis. Patient who presented with severe flank pain and haematuria. **(A)** A contrast-enhanced study showed a distal ureteric stone (arrow), causing hydronephrosis and hydroureter. **(B, C)** Note fluid outside the ureter, indicating likely rupture of the renal pelvis or ureter (arrow). **(D)** A delayed series confirmed rupture with contrast extravasation anterior to the renal pelvis (**D**, arrow). (CT images courtesy of Dr Damian Tolan, Consultant Radiologist, Leeds Teaching Hospitals, Leeds, UK.)

Differential diagnosis

When no renal tract calculi or secondary signs of acute renal tract pathology are detected, consider alternative diagnoses such as acute pyelonephritis (Fig. 4.43), appendicitis, pancreatitis, diverticulitis, perforation or adnexal pathology. Most acute abdominal pathologies will be apparent on non-contrast imaging, but the option is there to proceed with a post-contrast study if necessary to confirm the diagnosis.

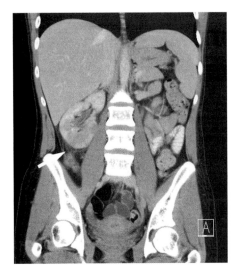

Figure 4.43: Acute pyelonephritis. Female patient who presented with right flank pain and fever. Coronal image shows low attenuation changes in a swollen lower pole right kidney along with perirenal stranding (arrow).

Acute reporting

- Identify and record the size and position of any urinary calculi.
- Look for signs of obstruction.
- Identify any secondary signs of acute renal compromise.
- If no urinary pathology is found, identify other abdominal pathology which might explain the patient's symptoms.

Recommended reading

Chowdhurya FU, Kotwalb S, Raghunathana G, Waha TM, Joyceb A, Irving HC. Unenhanced multidetector CT (CT KUB) in the initial imaging of suspected acute renal colic: evaluating a new service. *Clin Radiol* 2007;**62**:970–7.

Rucker CM, Menias CO, Bhalla S. Mimics of renal colic: alternative diagnoses at unenhanced helical CT. *Radiographics* 2004;**24**:S11–S33.

Acute abdomen: gynaecological causes

Summary

Protocol: Oral and IV contrast, full abdominal and pelvic bowel contrast, 2.5–5 mm collimation.

What to look for: Haemoperitoneum, ovarian enlargement, ovarian cysts, tubo-ovarian abscess, uterine fibroids.

Report: Confirm or exclude ovarian/uterine pathology and related complications.

In the setting of an acute abdomen, MDCT has a very limited role in the primary diagnosis of gynaecological pathology. CT may be requested if an initial pelvic ultrasound has been equivocal, but as ionizing radiation is an important consideration in women of reproductive age, the decision to perform CT should be carefully discussed with the referring clinicians. The possibility of pregnancy must be excluded in all cases. For potential gynaecological pathologies, ultrasound will generally be the initial investigation performed. MRI offers an alternative diagnostic option.

The common gynaecological causes of acute abdominopelvic pain include complicated ovarian cyst, ovarian torsion, pelvic inflammatory disease, uterine fibroid degeneration/torsion, ruptured ectopic pregnancy and postpartum complications.

Protocol and technique

Contrast enhancement: Oral and IV contrast. Imaging in portal venous phase with abdominal/pelvic bowel contrast. A reasonably full bladder is advantageous.

Collimation: 2.5–5 mm axial sections with coverage from diaphragm to symphysis. Coronal and sagittal reformats as required.

What to look for on CT

- Remember in females of reproductive age, a trace of free pelvic fluid is a common normal finding that should not be taken as an indicator of pelvic pathology. Deciding what represents a non-physiological volume of fluid is usually not difficult, but with smaller volumes, always keep an open mind that the findings could be within normal limits. Recognize pelvic fluid by detecting the classic CT appearance on axial sections of rectum posteriorly, urinary bladder anteriorly and ascites lying in-between these two structures. If the urinary bladder is almost empty, it can be difficult to decide what represents free fluid and what is due to partially collapsed bladder. Careful review is required to differentiate between the two.
- Always compare the density of any pelvic fluid with the density of unopacified urine in the adjacent bladder. Pelvic fluid of higher density than urine will generally indicate a haemoperitoneum. When present, look for a focal haematoma to identify a potential source for the haemoperitoneum.
- On unenhanced CT, be careful not to mistake the uterus for a mass-like pathology, especially if the uterine orientation is atypical or fibroids are present. On post-contrast imaging, the uterus enhances

strongly, which allows easy identification. If IV contrast is contraindicated, always consider the uterus as an explanation for a pelvic mass and confirm with the patient or the referring clinicians whether the uterus remains in situ or not.

■ Remember to carefully review the anatomy of both iliac fossae as pathologies originating outside the pelvis often track caudally into the adnexal territories and mimic primary gynaecological disease. It is always good practice to attempt to identify a normal appendix in the case of right-sided adnexal change. On the left, complicated diverticular disease may offer an alternative diagnosis.

Complicated ovarian cyst (Fig. 4.44)

■ The common complication is haemorrhage within the cyst. As unenhanced images are unlikely to be available as part of a survey type study, compare the density of the cyst content with other fluid-filled structures, such as the urinary bladder. Haemorrhagic fluid may layer within the cyst, giving high-density fluid–fluid levels.

■ Associated high-density ascites indicating haemoperitoneum along with pericyst haematoma are features of a ruptured cyst. Haematoma can be extensive and may obscure any recognizable cyst remnant.

■ Infected ovarian cysts are not commonly found as part of an acute abdomen assessment. If present, mural thickening and increased enhancement along with gas foci in the minority would be anticipated.

Ovarian torsion

■ Look for unilateral ovarian enlargement with obliteration of adjacent fat planes.

■ Congestion of parametrial vessels is a typical finding.

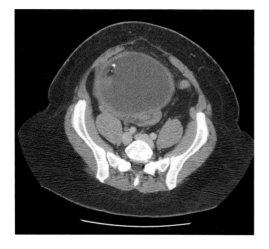

Figure 4.44: Dermoid cyst. Female patient who presented with acute lower abdominal pain. Mixed density mass showing cystic, solid, calcific and fatty elements enabled a CT diagnosis of adnexal dermoid. The pain at presentation suggested a complication and a torted ovarian dermoid was subsequently confirmed at laparotomy.

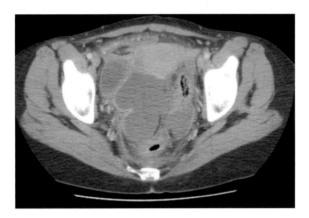

Figure 4.45: Pyosalpinx. Young female presented with lower abdominal pain and a vaginal discharge. Multifocal fluid-filled structures are seen within the pelvis. Operative findings confirmed a diagnosis of pyosalpinx.

- Pelvic ascites may be present.
- Look for uterine deviation to the side of the torted ovary.
- With the establishment of ovarian infarction, reduced or absent contrast enhancement, haematoma and/or gas formation are all signs that should suggest ischaemic compromise and the need for urgent surgical intervention.

Pelvic inflammatory disease

Pelvic inflammatory disease (PID) is an all-encompassing term covering a spectrum of pathologies of varying severity that develop as a complication of sexually transmitted disease. These include endometritis, salpingitis, tubo-ovarian abscess and pelvic peritonitis. Patients usually present with lower abdominal pain or adnexal pain, a vaginal discharge and raised inflammatory markers.

- In mild or early attacks, acute CT may be normal or the only finding may be low volume ascites.
- Tubo-ovarian abscess formation represents the more severe end of the PID spectrum and is generally secondary to the spread of infection from the lower genital tract. Look for a complex multiloculated adnexal mass, often associated with a fluid-filled distended Fallopian tube. Tubo-ovarian abscesses can be unilateral or bilateral (Figs 4.45, 4.46).

As with ovarian pathology, ultrasound is the imaging technique of choice. CT should not be used in the first instance but PID must be considered if CT has been performed for an alternative suspected clinical diagnosis and adnexal pathology is found.

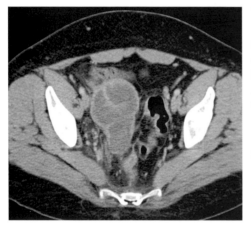

Figure 4.46: Ovarian abscess. Multicystic mass located in the right lower pelvis with minimal adjacent inflammatory changes. Presentation with pain and fever supported tubo-ovarian abscess which was confirmed at subsequent laparotomy. (CT image courtesy of Dr Andrea Sanderson, Consultant Radiologist, Pinderfield General Hospitals, Wakefield, UK.)

Uterine fibroids

Uterine fibroid complications do not commonly result in an acute abdomen.

- An uncomplicated fibroid uterus will be identified by uterine enlargement containing focal masses of varying number, size and morphology. These can be subserosal, intramural or submucosal in location. The periuterine tissues will be clean with preserved fat planes and no increase in physiological volumes of free fluid.
- Areas of low attenuation and poor contrast enhancement usually indicate liquefaction secondary to hyaline degeneration.
- Pedunculated fibroids are at risk of torsion and may present as an acute abdomen. Suspect when a juxtauterine mass is identified in a patient with a fibroid uterus. The findings can be very similar to those of ovarian torsion and differentiating between the two pathologies may be impossible, with the final diagnosis only being made at subsequent surgery.

Endometriosis

Endometriosis is the presence of endometrial-like tissue located outside the endometrial cavity. Endometrial deposits can be located in pelvic sites, such as the vagina and ovaries, or in more distant locations as diverse as laparotomy scars, the lung and spinal canal. Pelvic pain, classically cyclical, is the usual complaint with more acute presentations often related to secondary complications such as obstruction to bowel or the renal tract. Adhesions are a further recognized complication of the intraperitoneal inflammatory change associated with endometrial deposits.

- Ultrasound is the preferred method of imaging for pelvic presentations with magnetic resonance offering an alternative.
- Pelvic findings range from simple to complex cysts to solid masses.
- CT signs are non-specific with cysts of varying complexity involving ovaries or uterus among the commoner findings.
- Always consider a complication of endometriosis when unexplained bowel or renal tract pathology is found in females of appropriate age. However, the diagnosis is usually made at laparotomy or laparoscopy rather than by acute imaging.

Ruptured ectopic pregnancy

This remains the leading cause of first trimester maternal death. The classical presentation of abdominal pain, vaginal bleeding and an adnexal mass is only found in around 50% of cases. Diagnosis requires a positive beta-human chorionic gonadotrophin (HCG) test along with supporting imaging findings that include:

- An absent intrauterine gestation sac.
- A tubal gestation sac.
- Tubal haematoma.
- An adnexal mass with associated haemorrhagic fluid.

Ultrasound or magnetic resonance for the stable patient are the favoured imaging methods. A CT diagnosis of ectopic pregnancy generally follows an acute abdominal assessment for an alternative clinical diagnosis.

Postpartum complications

- CT is very unlikely to be the first-line approach to imaging a postpartum patient with acute abdominal symptoms unless bleeding is a likely clinical diagnosis.
- Look for excessive haematoma and signs of active contrast extravasation.
- Look for unexpected degrees of intrauterine debris that would suggest retained products (Fig. 4.47).
- Abscess formation is an unlikely complication, assuming a prior normal delivery and the absence of established pelvic inflammatory disease.
- Confirm uterine wall integrity to exclude perforation (in cases of surgical instrumentation). Perforation is usually associated with an enhancing parametrial collection.
- Look for signs of ovarian vein thrombosis.
- Omental infarction can rarely follow a difficult caesarian section.

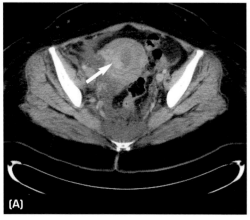 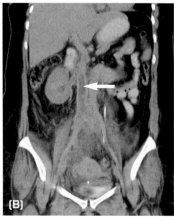

Figure 4.47: Complicated retained placenta. This patient presented with vaginal bleeding and abdominal pain following recent termination of pregnancy. **(A)** CT showed fluid within the uterine cavity and right lateral uterine wall hypervascularity (arrow). **(B)** CT also demonstrated a thrombosed ovarian vein extending to the inferior vena cava and right renal vein (arrow). Note the reduced right renal enhancement, indicating significant venous compromise. (CT images courtesy of Dr Damian Tolan, Consultant Radiologist, Leeds Teaching Hospitals, Leeds, UK.)

HELLP syndrome

- More common in pre-eclamptic patients.
- Look for haemoperitoneum.
- Pleuropericardial effusions and pulmonary oedema may be present.
- Look for subhepatic or intrahepatic haemorrhage.
- Look for active contrast extravasation and if found, urgent intervention is required.

Acute reporting

- Comment on the presence and extent of free fluid and make note of its density.
- Describe any mass or collection/abscess and suggest the likely origin.
- Look for asymmetrical enhancement of ovarian tissue, abnormal fibroid enhancement.
- If haematoma or haemoperitoneum present, carefully look for signs of contrast extravasation.

- Exclude or confirm pathology of either iliac fossa as an alternative diagnosis to primary pelvic disease.
- Remember that a normal CT does not exclude conditions such as pelvic inflammatory disease, ruptured ectopic pregnancy and ovarian torsion–detorsion.

Recommended reading

Bennett GL, Slywotzky CM, Giovanniello G. Gynecological causes of acute pelvic pain: spectrum of CT findings. Education exhibit. *Radiographics* 2002;**22**:785–801.
Potter AW, Chandrasekhar CA. US and CT evaluation of acute pelvic pain of gynecologic origin in nonpregnant premenopausal patients. *Radiographics* 2008;**28**:1645–59.

The postoperative abdomen

Summary

Protocol: Oral and IV contrast. Omit oral contrast if bowel obstruction is likely.

What to look for: Free fluid and gas in excess of what would be anticipated for that stage of the post-operative recovery: collections, abscess, retained surgical material, injury to adjacent organs: vascular complications. Decide if bowel obstruction or ileus. Identify renal tract compromise.

Reporting: Location and extent of fluid and gas. Document any collections/abscesses, their size and location, and any percutaneous drainage options.

Requests for imaging the postoperative abdomen is a common out-of-hours occurrence and as such, a basic knowledge of the commoner surgical procedures and their potential complications is a requirement for any radiologist involved in such imaging (see, for example, Figs 4.48–4.51). MDCT is ideally suited for this task as its speed and flexibility are major advantages for patients who are often unwell. Close clinicoradiological liaison to establish the exact nature of any surgical procedure performed is a must before any scanning commences.

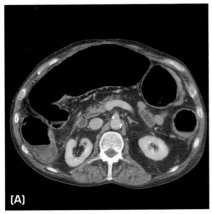
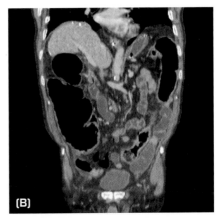

(A)   **(B)**

Figure 4.48: Pseudo-obstruction post reversal of ileostomy. (A) Axial and **(B)** coronal sections demonstrate a distended right colon and transverse colon with relatively collapsed distal descending and sigmoid colon. The caecal and proximal ascending colonic walls show worrisome thickening along with early pericaecal oedema. Compare these segments of colon with the hepatic flexure and transverse colon that show normal mural morphology. The caecal diameter measured 11 cm, indicating a need for urgent decompression. A flatus tube was subsequently passed with good clinical effect.

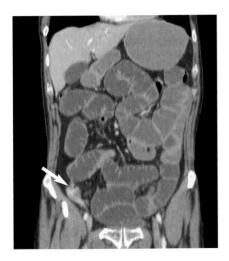

Figure 4.49: High-grade small bowel obstruction post anterior resection with covering loop ileostomy. Arrow identifies transition point, shown at subsequent laparotomy to be due to adhesions. This is an excellent illustration of why there is no need to routinely give oral contrast to patients with a high probability of small bowel obstruction. The fluid-filled small bowel provides excellent anatomical delineation.

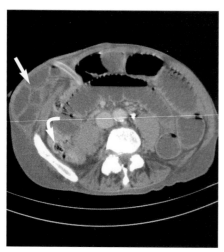

Figure 4.50: Small bowel obstruction. Post-laparoscopic anterior resection. Small bowel obstruction secondary to a loop of small bowel herniating through the right flank port site that had been inappropriately used for a drainage catheter. Note significantly dilated intra-abdominal small bowel loops with further dilated small bowel located outside the abdominal cavity (arrow) adjacent to the surgically placed drain. A small section of non-dilated caecum can be seen (curved arrow) adjacent to the iliac wing.

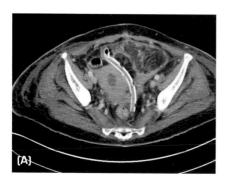
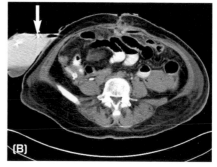

Figure 4.51: Drain related trauma. Recent subtotal colectomy complicated by persistent drainage of enteric content. **(A)** Conventional CT with oral contrast had not established a diagnosis. **(B)** A second series, following administration of rectal contrast, showed colonic contrast entering the drainage bag (arrow), confirming a colonic leak that was subsequently repaired at laparotomy. Assumed due to drain-related trauma. This is a good example of the selective use of colonic contrast.

Protocol & technique

Contrast enhancement: Oral and IV contrast. Omit oral contrast if bowel obstruction is likely.

Slice collimation: 2.5–5 mm axial reconstruction, coronal/sagittal reconstructions as required.

What to look for on CT

- Assess the volume of any free fluid and gas and decide if either is in excess of what might be expected for this stage of the postoperative recovery. Check the CT density of free fluid and identify any haemoperitoneum.
- Assess the abdominal wound: wound sepsis more commonly occurs during the second or third postoperative week. CT signs include collections of fluid and/or gas within the abdominal wall close to the surgical incision site. These can remain superficial or form fistulous tracks that extend into the peritoneal or retroperitoneal cavities.
- Assess the anastomosis: look for a larger volume of perianastomatic gas than expected for the stage of postoperative recovery, or increasing volumes on sequential studies. Identify a localized collection or abscess in the surgical bed, and extravasation of any bowel contrast (Figs 4.52, 4.53).
- Abscess formation: look for a well-circumscribed fluid collection with a peripherally enhancing rim. Gas will only be found in the minority. An abscess will typically impact on adjacent anatomy producing a mass effect. Simple non-infected fluid collections tend to mould around or invaginate between adjacent anatomical structures.
- Look for retained surgical materials such as swabs and surgical instruments. The scout film should be reviewed before the axial images are acquired.

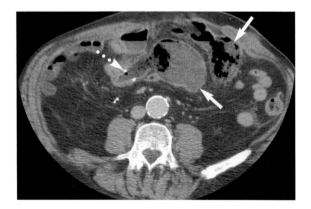

Figure 4.52: Anastomotic breakdown following extended right hemicolectomy. Multifocal perienteric collections (arrows) showing gas and fluid densities extending from the disrupted suture line (dotted arrow).

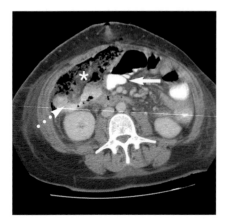

Figure 4.53: Anastomotic leak. Small bowel leak following resection of ischaemic small bowel. Axial image shows intraluminal small bowel contrast (arrow), extravasated extraluminal small bowel contrast (dotted arrow) and an abscess lying between the rectus and bowel (star).

Haemostatic agents placed during surgery to control haemorrhage can very much mimic abscess formation. Always consider this option. Surgeons rarely share this information, so enquiry may be necessary to avoid a mis-diagnosis.

Interventional aspects

CT-guided drainage of an intra-abdominal abscess or collection offers an alternative to ultrasound-guided drainage. CT has clear advantages in some postoperative abdomens when ileus, drainage catheters, and skin dressings may all compromise ultrasound access and adequate demonstration of the anatomy. Always ensure a safe route of access before placing any drainage catheter. Never deliberately cross the colon. Transgluteal drainage should be reserved for patients in whom no alternative means of pelvic drainage is possible and when it is necessary to temporize before surgery.

Acute reporting

- Confirm or discount whatever complication is suspected clinically.
- Document the distribution and size of any collections as well as suggesting any options for percutaneous drainage.
- Attempt to differentiate between obstruction and ileus.

Recommended reading

Gore R, Berlin J, Yaghmai V, Mehta U, Newmark GM, Ghahremani GG. CT diagnosis of postoperative complications. *Semin Ultrasound CT MRI* 2004;**25**:207–21.

Zissin R, Osadchy A, Gayer G. Computed tomography findings of early abdominal postoperative complications. *Can Assoc Radiol J* 2007; **58**:136–45.

5 Paediatrics

The acute paediatric abdomen

Summary

Protocol: Oral and intravenous (IV) contrast. Image in portal venous phase.

Look for: Causes of childhood abdominal pain, such as appendicitis, intussusception, mesenteric adenitis.

Report: Describe cause and severity of abdominal pain and complications.

Abdominal pain is one of the most frequently encountered complaints in the emergency room, but a child's inability to describe his or her symptoms combined with an equivocal clinical examination makes establishing a definite diagnosis difficult. While children share many of the common causes of abdominal pain with adults, they also have some less common causes that may be incidentally diagnosed on cross-sectional imaging ordered for an alternative clinical diagnosis, usually appendicitis.

Protocol and technique

Contrast enhancement: Omit the non-contrast examination to reduce the radiation dose. Administer IV contrast for a portal venous-phase acquisition, usually 50–60 s after bolus. Administer oral contrast based on weight, 1 h prior to scanning with half the initial volume given 15 min before scanning.

Slice collimation: 2.5–5 mm axial, reconstruction with coronal and sagittal reformats as necessary.

What to look for on CT

The commoner causes of acute abdominal pain in children include:

- Appendicitis.
- Intussusception.
- Mesenteric adenitis.
- Midgut volvulus.
- Meckel diverticulitis.
- Henoch–Schönlein purpura.
- Hydrometrocolopos.
- Pyelonephritis.
- Ovarian torsion.
- Cholecystitis.
- Pancreatitis.
- Gastroenteritis.
- Inflammatory bowel disease.
- Pneumonia.
- Splenomegaly from mononucleosis.

This section will concentrate on those diagnoses that are more commonly found in children. Appendicitis, cholecystitis, pancreatitis, gastroenteritis and inflammatory bowel disease are covered in Chapter 4.

Intussusception

- Location is commonly at or close to the caecum, but can be anywhere along the gastrointestinal tract, especially where there is a pathologic lead point or in cases where a long segment has telescoped.
- The bowel mass contains concentric rings of alternating high and low density.
- Mesenteric fat stranding usually accompanies the bowel mass.
- Look for a pathologic lead point, particularly in older children (Fig. 5.1). Although lead lesions are frequently present, these may not be readily appreciated on CT, with the final diagnosis only becoming apparent at laparotomy.
- Look for associated lymphadenopathy that might suggest mesenteric adenitis or lymphoma as a background aetiology.
- In later stages, if bowel necrosis/perforation develops, pneumoperitoneum, pneumatosis and portal venous gas may be seen.

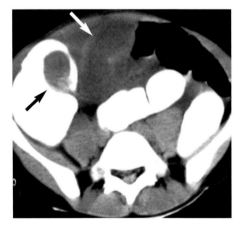

Figure 5.1: Meckel diverticulum leading to intussusception. A pedunculated soft tissue mass (black arrow) acts as the intussusceptum within the dilated contrast-filled caecum. This was proven to be a Meckel diverticulum at surgery. Note the fluid-filled loops of distal small bowel (white arrow). (CT image courtesy of Dr M Ines Boechat, Division of Paediatric Radiology, Department of Radiological Science, University of California, Los Angeles, USA.)

Interventional aspects: The barium/air-contrast enema is both diagnostic and therapeutic. If three attempts at reduction fail, surgery is required. Recurrence is most common in the following 72 h and occurs in 10–15% of patients.

Mesenteric adenitis

- A cluster of three or more lymph nodes measuring at least 5 mm in short axis in the right lower quadrant with a *normal* appendix.
- Further lymph nodes may be found throughout the mesentery.
- Lymphadenopathy may accompany appendicitis, so look for a normal appendix to exclude appendicitis.
- If the appendix is not seen, the diagnosis is made surgically.

Midgut volvulus

- The superior mesenteric venous and arterial relationship is reversed with the smaller superior mesenteric artery lying to the left of a larger superior mesenteric vein. This sign is neither sensitive nor specific and may be found in normal patients *without* malrotation. Oedematous bowel may be seen to swirl around the superior mesenteric vessels.
- Non-specific signs of ischaemic compromise include flaccid distension, pneumotosis and/or altered wall enhancement, perforation, pneumoperitoneum and portal venous air.
- A definitive diagnosis is made by an upper gastrointestinal contrast study, but in established cases the CT findings are usually diagnostic and emergency surgery is required to ensure preservation of bowel viability.

Meckel diverticulitis

- Often mimics appendicitis. Look for a blind-ending tubular structure with associated pericaecal soft tissue stranding, and in the presence of contained perforation, localized abscess formation.
- Secondary small bowel obstruction may be the only sign.
- Look for concomitant intussusception with findings as described above.

A Tc-99m pertechnetate scan is 90% accurate when a Meckel diverticulum contains ectopic gastric mucosa. The diverticulum will require surgical excision, usually with appendectomy performed at the same time.

Henoch–Schönlein purpura

A multisystem disease with a plethora of imaging abnormalities.

- **Pulmonary findings:**
  - ☐ Pleural effusion reflecting nephritic syndrome.
  - ☐ Interstitial infiltrates with subpleural reticulations.
- **Abdominal findings:**
  - ☐ 2% present with intussusception.
  - ☐ Non-specific lymphadenopathy.
  - ☐ Bowel wall oedema, haemorrhage or mucosal thumbprinting due to vasculitis of the splanchnic blood vessels.
  - ☐ Non-specific colitis.
- **Genitourinary abnormalities** include:
  - ☐ Renal oedema.
  - ☐ Scrotal wall oedema and skin thickening without underlying testicular/epididymal enlargement or hyperaemia.

Renal insufficiency may require dialysis or transplantation. Some patients undergo exploratory laparotomy because the abdominal symptoms may mimic an acute abdomen and can occur before the rash and renal insufficiency become established. Up to 50% of patients will recur, usually within the first 6 weeks, but this can be years later.

Pyelonephritis (Fig.5.2)

A clinical urinary tract infection with an equivocal urrinalysis may prompt an imaging request to rule out appendicitis, which can be clinically indistinguishable and may even show sterile pyuria on urinalysis.

- The affected kidney will be oedematous with poor corticomedullary differentiation.
- Enhancement may show a 'striated nephrogram' or focal areas of hyper- or hypo-density.
- A focal mass/swelling may mimic a primary renal or adrenal tumor, such as nephroblastoma or Wilms tumor.
- Perinephric fat stranding and/or possible perinephric fluid are secondary findings.

Be sure to recommend outpatient renal scintigraphy and renal ultrasound following resolution of the infection to exclude underlying vesicoureteral reflux.

Hydrometrocolpos/hydrocolpos

- The distended vaginal vault may displace the rectum, bowel, urinary bladder and/or uterus.
- With ureteral obstruction, the renal pelvis may become dilated.
- The uterus enhances and may also dilate. Dilatation may also involve the Fallopian tubes.

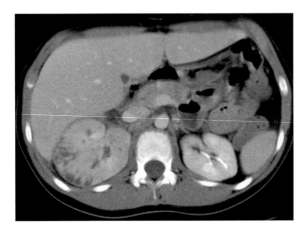

Figure 5.2: Pyelonephritis with abscesses. A 10-year-old boy who presented with fever and abdominal pain. The right kidney is enlarged with reduced cortical enhancement and multiple peripheral hypodense foci representing abscesses.

- The distending fluid may be of water density or higher density due to proteinacious debris and old blood products.
- Renal, anal, vertebral and/or cardiac anomalies are rare associations.

The uterus may demonstrate other developmental anomalies and ultrasound or MRI may be required to further evaluate these.

Ovarian torsion

Doppler ultrasound is the preferred examination. Some children may be initially referred for CT, particularly when appendicitis is the leading diagnosis and the institution does not routinely use ultrasound as the first-line technique for the diagnosis of appendicitis.

- The Fallopian tube is oedematous and dilated.
- The uterus typically deviated toward the affected side.
- The infarcted ovary does not enhance.
- Typically, torsion is a complication of an ovarian mass. The pathological ovary may show eccentric wall thickening with lack of enhancement of the internal solid components.
- Haemorrhagic infarction causes haemoperitoneum, mural thickening of the affected Fallopian tube and intratumoral haemorrhage within any associated ovarian mass.

This is a surgical emergency (to avoid ovarian infarction) and the patient should undergo urgent operative detorsion with removal of any associated mass.

Ovarian teratoma (Fig. 5.3)

Patients with ovarian teratoma may present with an abrupt onset of abdominal pain when tumoral haemorrhage or torsion occur. Ultrasound

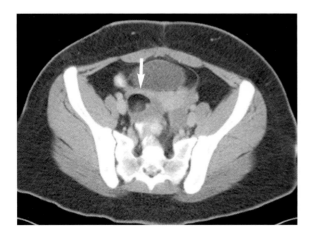

Figure 5.3: Right ovarian teratoma. A 15-year-old female with right lower quadrant abdominal pain. Note the fat-containing right adnexal mass (arrow), which is consistent with a teratodermoid.

is again the modality of choice, accepting that alternative clinical diagnoses may lead to a patient initially undergoing CT. These tumours contain tissue from all three embryologic germ cell layers.

- Fat, teeth, calcification and hair often predominate.
- Tumours may be septated and have a thickened capsular wall.
- Debris and fluid layering may be recognized within the cystic compartments.

Acute reporting

- For surgical abdomens, immediate discussion with the referring clinician is required.
- Carefully look for signs of perforation or ischaemic compromise to the bowel.
- Look for signs of severe dehydration or shock, such as a diminutive inferior vena cava.
- Lower lobe pneumonia may present as abdominal pain in children, so the included lower lung fields need to be evaluated.
- Splenomegaly may complicate conditions such as infectious mononucleosis with stretching of the capsule leading to significant abdominal pain. This may be the presenting complaint.

Deep neck infections in children

Infants with stridor and symptoms of infection usually are managed clinically because croup, exudative tracheitis and epiglottitis do not usually require CT for diagnosis. However, if retropharyngeal abscess is a likely diagnosis, cross-sectional imaging is required to evaluate the extent of disease and to determine if the infection will require surgical drainage.

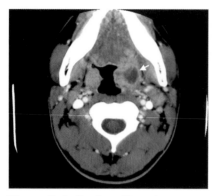

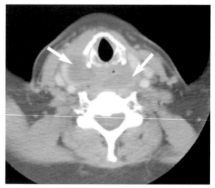

Figure 5.4: Peritonsillar abscess. This 19-year-old male had a history of multiple tonsillar infections. CT shows a rim-enhancing hypodensity deep to the left tonsillar pillar, indicating a drainable abscess (arrow). Note the associated narrowing and rightward displacement of the oropharynx. The vessels and carotid sheath are uninvolved. (CT image courtesy of Dr Noriko Salamon, Division of Paediatric Radiology, Department of Radiological Science, University of California, Los Angeles, USA.)

Figure 5.5: Retropharyngeal abscess. This 16-year-old patient had already undergone tonsillar abscess drainage and antibiotic treatment for streptococcus infection without symptom resolution. CT revealed a supraglottic retropharyngeal abscess within the pervertebral space (arrows). The aerodigestive tract and great vessels were involved. (CT image courtesy of Dr Noriko Salamon, Division of Paediatric Radiology, Department of Radiological Science, University of California, Los Angeles, USA.)

Differential diagnosis of stridor in children

- Epiglottitis.
- Croup.
- Bacterial tracheitis.
- Peritonsillar abscess (Fig. 5.4).
- Cervical lymphadenitis.
- Vascular rings/slings.
- Pseudothickening of the retropharyngeal soft tissues.
- Foreign body aspiration.

Retropharyngeal abscess (Fig. 5.5)

Infants typically are 6–12 months of age, although older children may also be affected. Antecedent otitis media, streptococcal pharyngitis, and/or viral upper respiratory infection will be elicited on history. Symptoms include stiff neck, stridor, dysphagia, trouble handling oral secretions and sudden onset of high fever.

What to look for on CT:

- The retropharyngeal soft tissues will be thickened with mass effect impinging on the airway.
- Associated soft tissue gas, when present, is a specific sign.
- The palatine tonsils are enlarged with increased contrast enhancement.
- Fat planes will be obliterated.
- Abscesses are typically hypodense with an enhancing rim.

Interventional aspects: In the absence of an abscess, management is medical with intravenous antibiotics. Abscesses require surgical drainage.

Acute reporting: When any signs of airway vulnerability are detected, contact the referring clinician immediately.

- Define abscess location, size and drainage options.
- Look for ancillary signs that have both surgical and prognostic implications:
  - ☐ Involvement of the carotid sheath.
  - ☐ Jugular venous thrombosis.
  - ☐ Extension of the inflammatory process to the mediastinum with or without evidence of mediastinitis. The latter has a high mortality.

Recommended reading

Craig FW, Shunk JE. Retropharyngeal abscess in children: clinical presentation, utility of imaging, and current management. *Pediatrics* 2003;**111**: 1394–98.

Daneman A, Navaro O. Intussusception. Part 2: An update on the evolution of management. *Pediatr Radiol* 2003;**34**:97–108.

Chang WL, Yang YH, Lin YT, Chiang BL. Gastrointestinal manifestations in Henoch-Schönlein purpura: a review of 261 patients. *Acta Paediatr* 2004;**93**:1427–31.

Daneman A, Navarro O. Intussusception. Part 1: a review of diagnostic approaches. *Pediatr Radiol* 2003;**33**:79–85.

Donnelly LF. *Diagnostic Imaging: Pediatrics*. Salt Lake City: Amirsys Inc, 2005.

Levy AD, Hobbs CM. From the archives of the AFIP: Meckel diverticulum: radiologic features with pathologic correlation. *Radiographics* 2004;**24**:565–87.

Navarro O, Daneman A. Intussusception 3: Diagnosis and management of those with an identifiable or predisposing cause and those that reduce spontaneously. *Pediatr Radiol* 2004;**33**:305–12.

Rao PM, Rhea JT, Novelline RA. CT diagnosis of mesenteric adenitis. *Radiology* 1997;**202**:145–9.

Rha SE, Byun JY, Jung SE, et al. Pictoral essay: Atypical CT and MRI manifestaions of mature ovarian cystic teratomas. *AJR Am J Roentgenol* 2004;**183**:743–50.

Rha SE, Byun JY, Jung SE, et al. CT and MR imaging features of adnexal torsion. *Radiographics* 2002;**22**:283–94.

Siegel MJ. *Pediatric Body CT*, 2nd edn. Philadelphia: Lippincott, Williams, & Wilkins, 2008.

6 Cardiac and Vascular

Recent developments in imaging hardware have lead to a rapid expansion in the use of CT for the investigation of vascular pathologies. Current spatial resolutions of 0.4–0.6 mm and improved temporal resolution (160 ms for 64-slice CT and 80 ms for dual-source CT) provide high-quality vascular imaging with very short examination times.

Although CT angiography (CTA) is typically read from the source data, good quality 3D reconstructions are essential for clear communication and demonstration of pathology to other specialists. In the emergency setting where time is of the essence, volume-rendered images and maximum intensity projections (MIPs) are most useful.

Vascular protocols are designed to maximize arterial contrast enhancement. The rate of contrast delivery and the volume of contrast used are the two parameters that can be varied to optimize the study. Ideally the scan time and the injection duration should be equal. A timing bolus can be used to monitor the transit of contrast. Alternatively, automated bolus triggering software can be used to optimize timing. No oral contrast should be given.

Aortic dissection

Summary

Protocol: Intravenous (IV) contrast. Triphasic scan. ECG gating (Fig. 6.1).

What to look for: An intimal dissection flap, a high density vessel wall indicating recent haemorrhage, whether the dissection involves the ascending aorta, descending aorta or both. Is the coeliac axis, superior mesenteric artery or renal arteries compromised by the dissection?

Report: Confirmation or exclusion of dissection, its location and extent, any associated vascular complications, and which vessels fill from the false lumen.

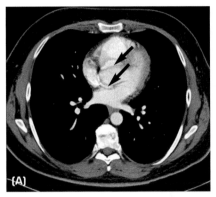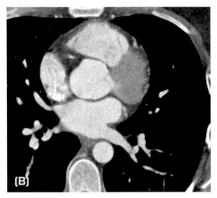

Figure 6.1: Aortic dissection: diagnostic pitfalls. A 52-year-old male who presented with suspected aortic dissection. **(A)** The initial CT, performed without cardiac gating, resulted in problematic linear artefact at the aortic root (arrows). **(B)** A repeat CT with ECG gating eliminated the artefact. The aortic root is normal.

Penetrating aortic ulcer, intramural haematoma and aortic dissection are now recognized as a spectrum of the same disease process. The traditional classification systems are now considered inadequate for appropriate management of aortic dissection. Both the de Bakey and the Stanford systems give anatomical information regarding the point of dissection, but do not address the effects of the injury. A descending thoracic aortic dissection crossing the abdominal visceral arteries is as life-threatening as an ascending aortic dissection.

Protocol and technique

As for blunt aortic trauma (see p 30), but continue scan to level of common femoral arteries. The entire aorta and iliac system should be

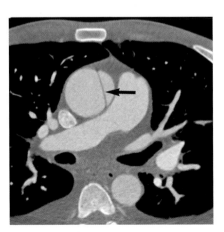

Figure 6.2: Aortic dissection. The axial section shows a linear dissection flap in the ascending aorta (arrow).

scanned. This allows visualization of the entire dissection and endovascular treatment planning if fenestration, aortic stenting or visceral arterial stenting is to be considered.

What to look for on CT

■ A **penetrating aortic ulcer** is ulceration of an atherosclerotic ulcer that extends through the intima and into the media.

■ This results in thinning of the wall of the aorta at the site of ulceration and once this occurs, bleeding into the media results in an **intramural haematoma**. The wall is now focally thickened and appears hyperdense on the non-contrast images if the bleeding is recent.

■ Further extension of the bleed eventually results in **aortic dissection**. This is seen as a linear filling defect extending for variable length through the vessel (Figs 6.2–6.4).

Interventional aspects

The point of origin of the dissection traditionally determines treatment options (see DeBakey and Stanford classifications). However, management is now best determined by the age of the dissection, the point of origin and any malperfusion complications.

Interventional radiology offers three management points in this disease: thoracic aortic stent grafting, branch vessel stent grafting, and fenestration of the intimal flap.

Acute complications, including rupture of the aorta, and cardiac complications require emergency treatment. A third group of complications, made up of malperfusion syndromes affecting the renal arteries, visceral

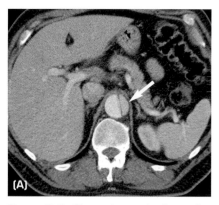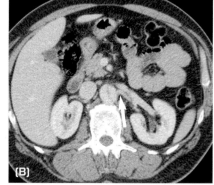

Figure 6.3: Thoracic aortic dissection extending into the abdomen. **(A)** Note the degree of contrast enhancement of the false lumen (arrow) is less than the true lumen. **(B)** The left renal artery is supplied by the false lumen (arrow).

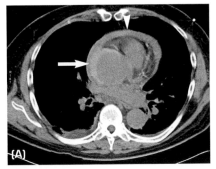 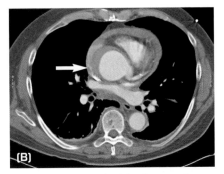

Figure 6.4: Aortic mural haematoma. Patient presented with chest pain and a clinical diagnosis of aortic dissection. **(A)** Unenhanced CT shows a dilated aortic root with a high-density crescentic intramural haematoma (arrow). Further high density is seen in the pericardial space, reflecting haemopericardium (arrowhead). **(B)** Arterial phase image reveals foci of vascular density (arrow) anterior to superior vena cava, indicating active haemorrhage. (CT images courtesy of Dr R Ratnalingam, Consultant Radiologist, Pinderfield General Hospital, Wakefield, UK.)

arteries and the lower limbs, can also be successfully treated. In this group, fenestration and branch stenting can be employed depending of the mechanism of the malperfusion.

Acute reporting

Document:

- The level of dissection and its extent.
- Branch vessels crossed by the dissection.
- Point of fenestration.
- Which vessels fill from the false lumen.

Coronary artery evaluation

Summary

Protocol: IV contrast. Non-contrast calcium score scan and arterial phase scan. ECG gating. Beta-blockade. Glyceryl trinitrate (GTN).

What to look for: Calcium score, variant anatomy, plaque assessment (site, hard/soft, ulceration, degree of stenosis).

Report: Calcium score, variant anatomy, vessel dominance, plaque assessment (site, hard/soft, ulceration, degree of stenosis), extracardiac disease.

The strength of coronary CTA is its high negative predictive value (almost 99%) and as such, it should be used in the emergency setting to exclude coronary artery disease in medium-to-low probability cases. A high probability cardiac chest pain (thrombolysis in myocardial infarction [TIMI] risk score ≥ 6) patient should go straight to angiography. Low probability cardiac chest pain (TIMI risk score 1–3) patients should have clinical assessment, clinical observation and laboratory testing. Medium probability cardiac chest pain patients (TIMI risk score 3–5), atypical chest pain, inconclusive electrocardiogram (ECG), exercise stress test (EST) or troponin profiles, have the greatest potential benefit from coronary CTA.

Protocol and technique

A coronary artery CT protocol either exists at your hospital or the service is not yet available. Each hospital will vary in its availability and its protocol, but the following basic approach is typical.

- Two sprays (800 μg) of sublingual GTN to dilate coronary vessels.
- Beta-blockade is used to bring the heart rate to <60 bpm. We use 15 mg of metoprolol IV in three divided doses as judged by rate response. Other institutions give 50 mg metoprolol the night before the test. If a dual source CT is used then rate control is not necessary below 100 bpm.
- A non-contrast coronary CT with calcium score is performed initially followed by a post-contrast coronary angiogram performed with bolus tracking for optimized timing.
- The raw data is then sent for post-processing. Post-processing is complex and needs much physician input. Images are reconstructed at different phases of the cardiac cycle, typically 30–40% for the right coronary artery (RCA), and 60–70% for the left main coronary artery (LMCA) and its branches. These phases are chosen based on visual assessment of the data collected. More than one phase is chosen per vessel. Each vessel is then reconstructed in a curved multiplanar reconstruction at these different phases.

What to look for on CT

- ***Coronary calcium score:*** This is given as a numerical score and relates to the risk of a coronary event occurring:

0	Minimal risk of adverse cardiac event
1–10	Mild risk of adverse cardiac event
11–100	Moderate risk of adverse cardiac event
101–400	High risk of adverse cardiac event
> 400	Extremely high risk of adverse cardiac event

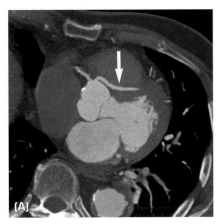
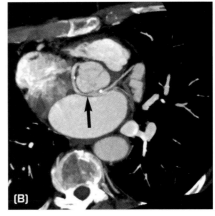

Figure 6.5: Coronary artery evaluation. (A) A 37-year-old male presented with recurrent chest pain on exertion. CT showed that the left coronary artery (arrow) passing between the aortic root and the pulmonary trunk. Referred to as a 'malignant' course, this can give rise to chest pain on exertion and sudden death. **(B)** A patient with an anomalous left coronary artery that shares a common trunk with the right coronary artery and passes between the aortic root and the left atrium (arrow). This is referred to as a 'benign' course. (CT images courtesy of Dr Edward Hoey, Specialist Registrar in Radiology, Leeds Teaching Hospitals, Leeds, UK.)

- **Vessel dominance:** The vessel which supplies the posterior descending artery and hence the AV node determines the dominance. In 80% the patent ductus arteriosus (PDA) arises from the RCA, 10% LCx, 10% codominant.
- **Aberrant anatomy:** Although there are many coronary artery variants, all of which are relevant if coronary intervention is planned, of most concern are 'malignant' variants where the aberrant vessel (RCA or LCA) passes between the pulmonary trunk and aortic root (Fig. 6.5).
- **Myocardial bridging:** The vessel (typically left anterior descending artery [LAD]) has an intramyocardial segment for part of its course, resulting in dynamic stenosis during systole.
- **Plaque assessment:** All vessels and their branches to 1.5 mm diameter need to be described. A detailed knowledge of coronary anatomy is necessary. Plaque is described as hard (calcified) or soft (non-calcified). The degree of stenosis/occlusion is described using the AHA system: non-obstructive <50%; significant >50–70%; critical 70–99%; total 100%. The length of the vessel segment involved must also be detailed. Lesions <10 mm are referred to as focal/discrete. Lesions >20 mm are referred to as diffuse/long. Vessel remodelling, the accumulation of fat/soft plaque within the wall, can be seen prior to luminal narrowing (Fig. 6.6).

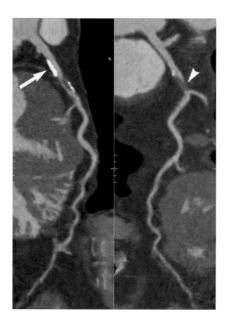

Figure 6.6: Coronary artery disease. Patient who presented with acute chest pain. Gated CT showed hard (arrow) and soft plaque (arrowhead) causing stenosis of the proximal part of the left anterior descending artery. The images displayed are orthogonal to each other.

- ■ *Coronary artery bypass graft (CABG) assessment:* In this setting it is important to commence the scan from the base of the neck so as to include the internal mammary arteries and their origins. Both internal mammary artery grafts and saphenous vein grafts are well assessed by CTA. The run-off native vessels are typically poorly demonstrated due to heavy arterial calcification.
- ■ *Diagnostic pitfalls:* CT coronary angiography must be read with a detailed understanding of the performance limitations of the hardware used as well as the limitations imposed on the study by the disease process.
  - ☐ **Heavy focal calcification** can obscure the vessel lumen and result in overcalling the degree of stenosis. The distribution of calcium is as important in determining image quality as total calcium score. Some centres advocate that coronary angiography is of limited value if the calcium score is very high (>800). However, in our experience, if it is widely distributed throughout the coronary vasculature, then worthwhile diagnostic images can still be obtained even with scores >1000.
  - ☐ In the setting of existing **coronary artery stents,** intrastent patency cannot be accurately assessed.
  - ☐ **Movement artefacts** can cause considerable diagnostic confusion and experience helps to identify these. If caused by a specific beat, then this can be removed from the original dataset and the images reconstructed again.

- **Extracardiac disease:** Numerous extracardiac pathologies can be seen within the dataset including breast and lung carcinoma, liver metastases, lung fibrosis, etc. The dataset must be looked at on bone, lung and mediastinal windows, and all abnormalities detailed.

Differential diagnosis

Acute aortic syndrome and pulmonary embolism are the main differentials and both are discussed below.

Acute reporting

- Calcium score.
- Variant anatomy.
- Vessel dominance.
- Plaque assessment (site, hard/soft, ulceration, degree of stenosis).
- Extracardiac disease.

Pulmonary artery evaluation

Summary

Protocol: IV contrast. Pulmonary arterial phase scan.

What to look for: Focal expansion of vessel, central filling defect, ground-glass opacification, unenhancing consolidation, right heart strain.

Report: Site, size and number of emboli.

Pulmonary embolism is a common clinical condition caused by a clot in the pulmonary artery or its branches. In most cases it is not fatal, but it is a leading cause of hospital death. It is most commonly caused by embolism of clot from a deep venous thrombosis of the lower limbs. If anticoagulation is withheld after negative CT pulmonary angiogram (CTPA), the risk of an adverse event is 1–3%.

Protocol and technique

Contrast enhancement: A contrast-enhanced CT is performed through the lungs with the contrast bolus timed to maximize the pulmonary arterial enhancement. 100 ml IV contrast ideally given at 5 ml/s. Try and avoid the use of small peripheral hand veins wherever possible.

Slice collimation: 1–1.5 mm axial section reconstruction.

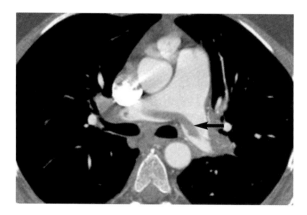

Figure 6.7:
Pulmonary embolism.
Arrow shows a large saddle embolus at the bifurcation of the main pulmonary artery.

What to look for on CT

- Findings on CT can be grouped into direct visualization of thrombus within the artery, the effect on the lung parenchyma and resultant cardiac strain.
- Findings relating to the pulmonary artery include focal expansion of the vessel and the presence of a central filling defect. When eccentric, this defect appears as a convex interface with the contrast. If the vessel is imaged in its horizontal plane, the contrast appears as parallel lines separated by the central thrombus (the tram track sign). If the vessel is orthogonal, it is seen as a central defect with a surrounding rim of contrast (rim sign) (Figs 6.7, 6.8).
- Now change the windows to view the parenchyma. Parenchymal signs include wedge-shaped ground-glass opacification, consolidation and unenhancing consolidation.
- Cardiovascular findings outside the pulmonary artery are predominantly those of increased right heart strain and include right ventricular enlargement, but not hypertrophy, and bowing of the interventricular septum. A patent foramen ovale should also be looked for as this places the patient at risk of paradoxical embolism.

Differential diagnosis

Aside from the obvious clinical differentials, the main imaging differential is chronic pulmonary embolus. In this situation the clot appears flat or concave with central contrast. Not infrequently, it is impossible to confidently differentiate between acute and chronic emboli. Flow artefacts can be problematic but are betrayed by the unclear edges to the clot. Coronal and sagittal reformatted images can help at times of diagnostic uncertainty, particularly where branching vessels can mimic emboli on axial images.

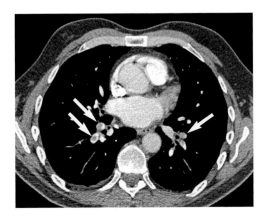

Figure 6.8: Pulmonary embolism. Filling defects in segmental branches of both pulmonary arteries indicate multiple emboli.

Acute reporting

Describe:

- Site, size and number of emboli.
- Complications such as pulmonary infarction and increased right heart strain.

Triple rule-out scan

The triple rule-out scan is designed to assess the patient for coronary arterial, pulmonary arterial and aortic disease in one scan. Some technical difficulties exist in maximizing image quality. This is particularly true for scanners with smaller detector banks (4, 16 and 40 slice). The advent of dual source multidetector CT (MDCT) has greatly reduced these problems and further advances, such as 256-slice MDCT will no doubt further improve image quality. However, high contrast within the aorta inherently degrades image quality in the pulmonary artery and vice versa. At present the triple rule-out scan has not been perfected; this is very much work in progress.

Infected (mycotic) aneurysms (Fig. 6.9)

Imaging features of inflammatory aneurysms include a lobulated or saccular configuration typically occurring in a vascular tree with little sign of generalized atheromatous change elsewhere. The aneurysm wall often displays prominent mural thickening, and perianeurysmal oedema or soft tissue extension may be found. Rarely gas foci can be identified in the aneurysm wall. Endovascular stent–graft repair is performed in selected cases as an alternative to open repair.

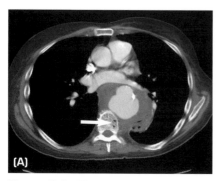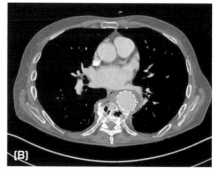

Figure 6.9: Mycotic aneurysm. (A) Saccular aneurysm formation with striking mural thickening. Note the foci of air in the adjacent vertebral body (arrow). This combination of CT signs should alert the reader to the possibility of an inflammatory aetiology. The aneurysm was treated by endovascular stenting. **(B)** A follow-up CT showed an interval improvement in the aneurysm appearances but a significant deterioration in the secondary involvement of the spine. (CT images courtesy of Dr S Puppala, Consultant Radiologist, Leeds General Infirmary, Leeds, UK.)

Penetrating atherosclerotic ulcer (Fig. 6.10)

This occurs when ulceration of an atherosclerotic plaque leads to penetration of the elastic lamina, and results in haematoma formation within the media of the aortic wall. On CT, the ulcer may be seen as a focal contrast bulge with adjacent mural haematoma. These changes are often best appreciated on sagittal reformatted images. Rupture or other life-threatening complications are uncommon but patients must be followed up particularly during the first month after the initial diagnosis. Surgical treatment may become necessary in cases where there is progression of intramural haematoma on follow-up imaging, clinical signs of impending rupture, an inability to control pain or significant blood pressure changes.

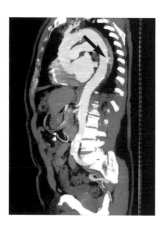

Figure 6.10: Penetrating aortic ulcer. Patient who presented with chest pain. Sagittal reformat of an arterial phase CT showing a contained contrast bulge in the posterior thoracic aortic wall indicating a penetrating ulcer (arrow). Note the associated acute mural haematoma.

Abdominal aortic aneurysm

Summary

Protocol: IV contrast. Triphasic scan.

What to look for: Retroperitoneal haematoma, discontinuity of aortic wall, intramural haemorrhage.

Report: Size of aneurysm, site (juxtarenal, infrarenal), degree of rupture/threatened rupture.

An abdominal aortic aneurysm is a localized dilatation of the aorta involving all three layers of the vessel wall. The risk of rupture increases with increasing size. Patients with abdominal pain and a large aneurysm but no frank rupture pose a diagnostic dilemma.

Protocol and technique

- Unenhanced CT through the abdomen and pelvis with 3 mm collimation.
- Bolus-tracked CTA of the abdomen and pelvis with 1 mm collimation.
- Delayed portal-venous (80 s) phase CT of abdomen and pelvis at 5 mm collimation.
- Contrast injection of 90 ml at 5 ml/s.

What to look for on CT

Rupture: Most ruptures manifest as retroperitoneal haematoma accompanied by an abdominal aortic aneurysm.

- Periaortic blood may extend into the perirenal space, pararenal space or both (Fig. 6.11).
- Extension into the psoas muscles and the peritoneal cavity may be seen with intraperitoneal haemorrhage, and is an immediate or a delayed finding.
- Discontinuity of the aortic wall or a focal gap in otherwise continuous circumferential wall calcifications may localize the point of rupture.

If the clinical question is simply one of confirmation or exclusion of aortic rupture, a non- contrast study alone may be all that is required for immediate management purposes. Increasingly, a full 'stent' protocol is performed during the acute study to fully evaluate the management options available.

Impending or contained rupture: This is difficult to identify at the best of times. There is usually a delay of several hours between acute

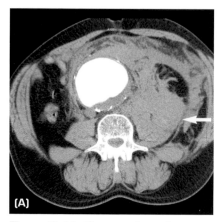 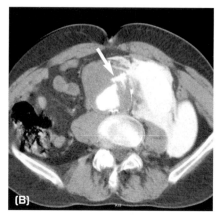

Figure 6.11: Ruptured aortic aneurysm. Two different patients presenting with back pain and in whom CT confirmed a ruptured abdominal aortic aneurysm. **(A)** Extensive retroperitoneal haematoma (arrow) but no active contrast leak at the time of the study. **(B)** Major contrast extravasation is shown (arrow). Both cases illustrate the typical retroperitoneal distribution of post-rupture haematoma. Local vascular surgical/interventional radiology practice will dictate whether intravenous contrast is given. In some centres, a limited non-enhanced study is all that is required. The signs of aneurysm rupture are rarely subtle. (CT images courtesy of Dr D Shaw, Consultant Radiologist, Pinderfield General Hospital, Wakefield, UK.)

intramural haemorrhage and frank extravasation into the periaortic soft tissues. This allows a window of opportunity for the patient and the clinician.

- Imaging features suggestive of impending rupture or instability include increased aneurysm size, a low thrombus-to-lumen ratio and haemorrhage into the mural thrombus.
- A peripheral crescent-shaped area of hyperattenuation within an abdominal aortic aneurysm represents an acute intramural haemorrhage. A small amount of periaortic blood may be mistaken for adenopathy, bowel or periaortic fibrosis.
- The contour of the aneurysm sac should also be looked at in detail. Draping of the posterior aspect of the aneurysm sac over the vertebrae is associated with a contained rupture.

Differential diagnosis

Remember any cause of acute abdominal pain, including pancreatitis, appendicitis, renal colic and small bowel obstruction, can present with a similar clinical picture.

Interventional aspects

Traditionally, emergency surgical repair is the primary treatment, although some centres provide emergency endovascular stent grafting for selected patients.

Acute reporting

Describe:

- Site and size of aneurysm.
- Degree of rupture/threatened rupture.
- Extent of the associated vascular disease and complications.

Gastrointestinal bleed

Summary

Protocol: IV contrast. Triphasic scan.

What to look for: High attenuation material in gut lumen, intraluminal contrast extravasation, underlying aetiology.

Report: Site of haemorrhage, arterial territory and variant anatomy.

Recently MDCT has become the first-line imaging modality for gastrointestinal bleeding, especially for the lower gastrointestinal tract. An upper gastrointestinal bleed is defined as haemorrhage proximal to the ligament of Treitz. It represents 70% of gastrointestinal bleeds and 75% will cease spontaneously. A lower gastrointestinal bleed, defined as haemorrhage occurring distal to the ligament of Treitz, represents 30% of gastrointestinal bleeds. Up to 80% of these will cease spontaneously. MDCT can detect bleeding rates as low as 0.3 ml/min.

Protocol and technique

No oral contrast should be given so that any positive contrast within the bowel lumen will be the result of extravasation. The initial non-contrast (5 mm sections) series is followed by an arterial phase (1–1.5 mm) and then a portal-venous phase (2.5–5 mm), with each phase covering the abdomen and pelvis.

It is important to ensure that the entire bowel is imaged, including the rectum. Imaging is best performed when the patient is actively bleeding and as such these patients are inherently unstable when they are being scanned. Active fluid resuscitation can be ongoing during the scan.

What to look for on CT

Haemorrhage: Fresh blood appears as high attenuation material within the bowel lumen. It is necessary to compare unenhanced images with enhanced images. As already mentioned, positive contrast appearing within the bowel after contrast injection represents extravasation

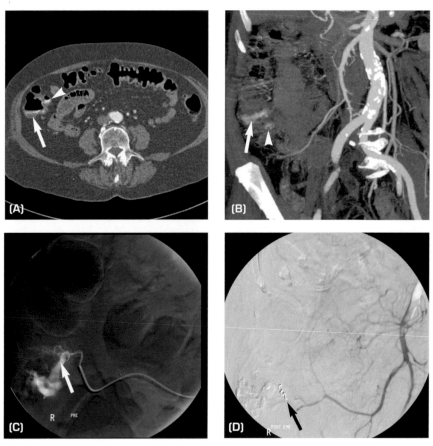

Figure 6.12: Colonic bleeding. Patient who presented with lower gastrointestinal haemorrhage. **(A)** Axial and **(B)** coronal CT performed during the arterial phase of contrast enhancement showed contrast accumulating within the ascending colon just above the ileocaecal valve (arrows). Note further contrast layering in a caecal diverticulum (arrowheads). **(C)** Angiography confirmed active extravasation from a branch of the ileocaecal artery (arrow) that was then **(D)** treated successfully by coil embolization (arrow). (CT and angiography images courtesy of Dr Ruth England and Dr Tony Nicholson, Consultant Radiologists, Leeds Teaching Hospitals, Leeds, UK.)

and is diagnostic of haemorrhage. When active extravasation is seen it may appear linear, jet-like, swirled, pooled or ellipsoid. Look for increasing contrast accumulation on the later phase images (Fig. 6.12). When haemorrhage is detected, attempts should be made to establish an aetiology, e.g. diverticulae or carcinoma. Angiodysplasia, a common cause of gastrointestinal bleeding, has no diagnostic features on CT.

Always document the vascular territory in which the bleed occurs as this will aid both surgical and endovascular planning as necessary.

Differential diagnosis

Pre-existing non-haemorrhagic high attenuation material in the gut lumen may be seen.

Interventional aspects

The increasing use of CT to localize the site of bleeding has resulted in a shorter procedure time, less contrast, less radiation exposure and faster catheterization of the bleeding vessel. Variant vascular anatomy can be demonstrated prior to intervention. CTA has also been shown to result in fewer negative/unnecessary conventional angiograms, as well as helping triage patients to endoscopy, interventional embolization or surgery.

Acute reporting

Describe:

- Site of haemorrhage.
- Arterial territory.
- Variant anatomy.

Limb angiography

Summary

Protocol: IV contrast. Triphasic scan.

What to look for: acute ischaemia (abrupt cut-off with no collaterals or distal filling); trauma (intimal tear, pseudoaneurysm, extravasation, AV fistula).

Report: Site and degree of injury, degree of distal compromise.

In the emergency setting there are two broad indications for CTA of the limbs: **acute limb ischaemia** and **limb trauma**, whether caused by motor vehicle accident, gun shot or stab injury.

Within the trauma subgroup, the clinical indications are broad and include diminished but appreciable pulse, excessive non-pulsatile bleeding, large non-expanding haematoma, major neurological/nerve deficit, an unappreciable pulse in an ischaemic extremity, absence of pulse with no definable trajectory from a single bullet, floating knee with a combined ipsilateral femoral–tibial fracture and a wound in proximity to a vessel.

Protocol and technique

Non-contrast, arterial phase and venous phase CTs are necessary for a complete examination but an arterial phase CT may be all that is needed if there is no clinical concern for venous injury. With modern systems, post-processing is a speedy exercise, allowing the findings to be displayed in an optimum manner for almost immediate clinicoradiological discussion.

What to look for on CT

- *Acute ischaemia:* Sudden abrupt cut-off with central thrombus, absent/poorly developed collaterals with or without reconstitution of distal vasculature. In chronic ischaemia collaterals are well developed with distal reconstitution of the run-off.
- *Trauma:* In order to visualize an intimal tear, use wide windows. Tears appear as a linear intravascular filling defect extending for a variable length. In addition, thrombus may be seen in association with the tear. A pseudoaneurysm appears as a well-circumscribed, rounded bulge contained within the adventitial covering. Less commonly, active extravasation may be seen. This typically looks like an irregular collection of contrast or may extravasate freely into adjacent tissues without forming a clear collection. Look for early venous filing which is diagnostic of an arteriovenous fistula. The extent of any perivascular haematoma should also be noted and a projectile tract or shrapnel within 5 mm of the neurovascular bundle should raise suspicion of occult vascular injury.
- *Pitfalls:*
  - In the setting of trauma, venous injury can be missed if a delayed venous phase is not acquired. As such, a separate protocol for acute ischaemia and trauma should exist.
  - Beam hardening and streak artefact caused by high-attenuation metal fragments can result in significant image degradation and render the adjacent area non-diagnostic.

☐ Vessel spasm can simulate occlusion.

☐ Technical factors may also result in a suboptimal study. For example, when assessing diseased arterial run-off, the scanner may overtake the contrast bolus, resulting in unopacified vessels distally.

Acute reporting

■ Site and degree of injury, degree of distal compromise.

■ Complications of trauma such as active contrast extravasation and perivascular haematoma, intimal tear, arteriovenous fistula and pseudoaneurysms.

Recommended reading

Flukinger T, White CS. Multidetector computed tomography in the evaluation of chest pain in the emergency department. *Semin Roentgenol* 2008;**43**:136–44.

Gaxotte V, Cocheteux B, Haulon S, et al. Relationship of intimal flap position to endovascular treatment of malperfusion syndromes in aortic dissection. *J Endovasc Ther* 2003;**10**:719–27.

Romano S (ed). Vascular emergencies. *Eur J Radiol* 2007;**64**:1–160.

Zimmet JM, Miller JM. Coronary artery CTA: imaging of atherosclerosis in the coronary arteries and reporting of coronary artery CTA findings. *Tech Vasc Interv Radiol* 2006;9:218–26.

7 Acute Neuroradiology

Subarachnoid haemorrhage

Summary

Protocol: Non-contrast imaging. CT cerebral angiogram to look for culprit aneurysm.

What to look for: Blood filling the subarachnoid spaces. Possible aneurysm.

Report: Confirm subarachnoid haemorrhage. Discuss with neurointerventionalist.

Subarachnoid haemorrhage refers to bleeding in the CSF space between the arachnoid and pia mater. In the non-trauma situation, subarachnoid haemorrhage typically results from rupture of a berry aneurysm but less commonly may be secondary to vascular anomalies of the spinal cord and meninges, coagulopathies, drug abuse and malignancy.

Protocol and technique

Contrast enhancement: Non-contrast CT brain, followed by cerebral angiography.

Slice collimation: 5 mm for non-contrast study; 0.625 mm acquisition for CT cerebral angiogram to allow the generation of high-quality multiplanar reformats.

What to look for on CT (Figs 7.1, 7.2)

- Carefully evaluate the cerebrospinal fluid (CSF) spaces. Subarachnoid haemorrhage is typically found in the interhemispheric fissure, suprasellar cistern, Sylvian fissure and perimesencephalic regions of the brain.
- Look for a causative berry aneurysm on the CT cerebral angiogram. Comment on its location, size and relationship to the parent vessel.

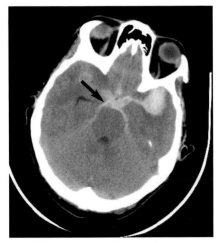

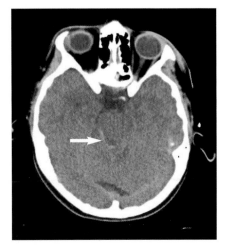

Figure 7.1: Subarachnoid haemorrhage. Non-contrast axial section through the mid-brain demonstrating high-density subarachnoid haemorrhage in the stellate (suprasellar) cistern (arrow). The concentration of blood in the left Sylvian fissure suggests this is the most likely site of a ruptured aneurysm.

Figure 7.2: Subarachnoid haemorrhage. There is effacement of the basal cisterns with subarachnoid haemorrhage in the right ambient cistern (arrow).

- Look for evidence of a vascular malformation or bleeding neoplasm (primary or secondary).
- Look for signs of mass effect: subfalcine herniation, uncal herniation at the tentorial hiatus and coning at the foramen magnum.

Differential diagnosis

Perimesencephalic haemorrhage in the setting of a 'normal' CT cerebral angiogram may represent a venous rather than an arterial bleed. These are associated with a better prognosis.

Interventional aspects

Early treatment is crucial and once the diagnosis is made, prompt discussion is required with the neurosurgeon and neurointerventionalist. Treatment options and the timing of any procedure will depend on local practices and expertise. The risk of re-rupture is the primary concern at this stage.

Acute reporting

- Confirm the presence and location of the subarachnoid haemorrhage.
- Identify any culprit aneurysm on CT cerebral angiogram.
- Liaise with local clinicians and neurosurgical centre.

Recommended reading

Tomandl BF, Köstner NC, Schempershofe M, et al. CT angiography of intracranial aneurysms: a focus on postprocessing. *Radiographics* 2004; **24**:637–55.

van Gijn J, Rinkel GJ. Subarachnoid haemorrhage: diagnosis, causes and management. *Brain* 2001;**124**:249–78.

Subdural haematoma

Summary

Protocol: Non-contrast imaging.

What to look for: Subdural haematoma.

Report: Confirm and describe secondary effects.

A subdural haematoma refers to blood in the space between the dura and arachnoid linings of the brain. Usually this follows stretching and tearing of the bridging cortical veins in this potential space due to sudden velocity changes. As such, a definite history of trauma may not be present, especially in the elderly. CT findings are characteristic and guide acute management.

Protocol and technique

Contrast enhancement: Non-contrast examination.

Slice collimation: 5 mm or less.

What to look for on CT (Figs 7.3–7.6)

- High-density blood spreading over the surface of the cerebral hemisphere in convex or concave shapes, unrestricted by suture linings.
- Signs of mass effect.
- In the anaemic patient, acute subdural haemorrhage may appear isodense to brain. In such cases, careful windowing is required to ensure the sulci extend to the cortical margin.

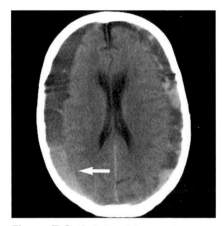

Figure 7.3: Subdural haematoma.
Bilateral convexity collections. A case of acute on chronic subdural haematoma. Note the characteristic dependent layering of acute blood (arrow).

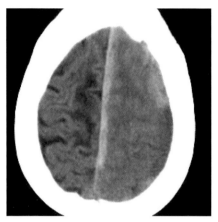

Figure 7.4: Subdural haematoma.
Extensive left-sided acute subdural haemorrhage. Note the parafalcine high-density change with effacement of the left sulcal pattern.

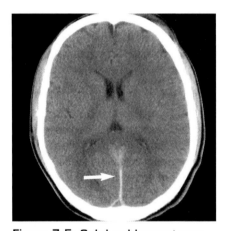

Figure 7.5: Subdural haematoma.
High density along the posterior aspect of the falx cerebri may be the only abnormal finding in an acute subdural haematoma (arrow).

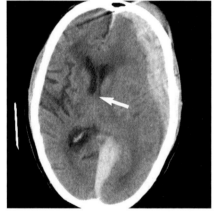

Figure 7.6: Subdural haematoma
exerting significant mass effect with large left frontotemporal convexity and left parieto-occipital parafalcine components. Note the contralateral midline shift (arrow).

Differential diagnosis

Trauma, coagulopathies, bleeding neoplasms, including surface or meningeal metastases, and arteriovenous malformations can all cause subdural haemorrhage.

Interventional aspects

Any subdural collection needs urgent discussion with the neurosurgeons to arrange decompression.

Acute reporting

- Confirm subdural haematoma; describe its location, extent and maximum width.
- Describe any secondary effects on surrounding tissues.

Extradural haematoma

Summary

Protocol: Non-contrast imaging.

What to look for: Extradural haematoma. Skull fracture.

Report: Confirm and describe any secondary effects.

Extradural haematoma refers to blood located between the periosteal and meningeal layers of the dural lining. Over 90% of cases are associated with traumatic injury to the middle meningeal artery.

Protocol and technique

Contrast enhancement: Non contrast imaging.

Slice collimation: 5 mm or less.

What to look for on CT (Fig. 7.7)

- Typically, a biconvex high-density collection (as the dura is firmly attached to the sutures). Fractures through a suture may breach the dural lining, resulting in less typical configurations.
- The grey–white interface is displaced away from the calvarium.
- Look carefully at the density of the haematoma. Active bleeding should be considered when areas of increased and decreased density with a whirling pattern are identified.
- Look for secondary herniation and pressure effects.
- Look for associated vault fracture on bone window
- Extradural haematoma may show delayed presentation following injury or may extend over time. As such, repeat and delayed imaging must be considered in all patients who show unexpected clinical deterioration.

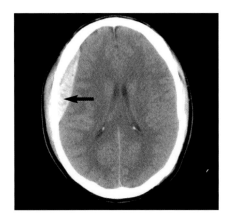

Figure 7.7: Extradural haematoma. Typical appearances of an acute extradural haematoma. Note the biconvex high-density haematoma (arrow) with mass effect on the underlying frontal lobe.

Differential diagnosis

Metastatic deposits extending from the skull vault may simulate extradural haematoma.

Interventional aspects

Extradural haematoma is a potentially lethal intracranial event and every case should be urgently discussed with the referring clinician with a view to urgent neurosurgical intervention.

Acute reporting

- Confirm the presence of an extradural haematoma.
- Comment on fractures if any.
- Is there evidence of active bleeding?
- Are there bilateral haematomas?
- Have neurosurgeons been alerted?

Recommended reading

Mayer S. NICE recommends greater use of CT imaging for head injuries. *BMJ* 2003;**326**:1414

Ischaemic stroke

Summary

Protocol: Non-contrast imaging.

What to look for: Early signs of infarct; exclusion of haemorrhage.

Report: A normal scan should be followed up with CT perfusion study and CT angiography.

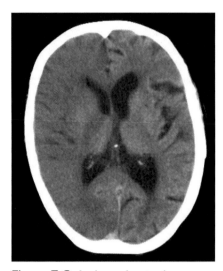 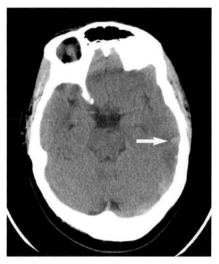

Figure 7.8: Ischaemic stroke.
Extensive infarction involving the right middle cerebral artery (MCA), posterior cerebral artery (PCA) and anterior cerebral artery (ACA) territories.

Figure 7.9: Haemorrhagic infarct.
An example of venous haemorrhagic infarct, which is typically cortical in location and may be associated with venous sinus thrombosis (arrow).

Multidetector CT (MDCT) has an established role in the early diagnosis of stroke. The primary objectives of early CT in the stroke patient are the exclusion of haemorrhage and the detection of early signs of infarction (Figs 7.8, 7.9). Non-enhanced CT has its limitations. It cannot distinguish between reversible and irreversible damage, a distinction that is crucial to the management of an acute brain attack. This distinction is best made by a CT perfusion study. CT angiography (CTA) will enable the evaluation of extra- and intra-cranial arteries for stenoses or occlusion. Urgent and appropriate intervention can then be planned for the patient.

Protocol and technique

Contrast enhancement: Non-contrast examination followed by CT perfusion study. Protocol depends on CT manufacturer, but typically 125 ml contrast given at 4 ml/s, the lower section to cover the basal ganglia. If negative for haemorrhage, CTA (C5 to vertex) is required.

Slice collimation: 5 mm for non-contrast CT and CT perfusion; 0.625 mm for CTA

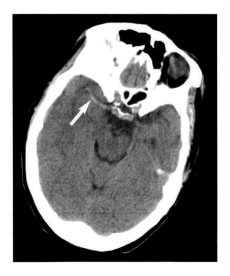

Figure 7.10: Ischaemic stroke. An example of the 'dense middle cerebral artery (MCA)' sign. The right MCA appears hyperdense (arrow) on this non-contrast CT due to intravascular thrombus.

What to look for on non-contrast CT

- In hyperacute stroke, the scan may appear normal on conventional unenhanced CT.
- One of the earliest signs of stroke is obscuration of the lentiform nucleus that is supplied by the lenticulostriate branches of the middle cerebral artery (MCA) (end-vessels, and therefore prone to ischaemia).
- Dense MCA (representing occlusion by a fresh thrombus); insular ribbon sign. The insular cortex is prone to ischaemic damage as it lies in the watershed area between the MCA and anterior cerebral artery (ACA) territory (Fig. 7.10).
- These signs may develop within 2 h of acute ischaemic insult.
- More established infarction will appear as hypodense areas in the affected vascular territory (Fig. 7.11).

What to look for on CT perfusion

Two important values that need evaluating on CT perfusion studies are cerebral blood flow (CBF) and cerebral blood volume (CBV). Modern scanners have automated programmes to assist with decision making in this situation. These terms have been explained below:

Cerebral blood flow: May be normal (50–60 mL/100 g/min) or reduced.
- 60% flow (moderate reduction) refers to oligaemic tissue that will probably survive.
- 30–60% flow (marked reduction) refers to tissue at risk that is potentially salvageable by reperfusion techniques.

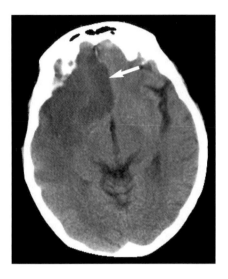

Figure 7.11: Ischaemic stroke. Ischaemic brain damage can display local mass effect due to associated cytotoxic oedema. In this case there is a right middle cerebral artery (MCA) territory infarct with midline shift (arrow).

■ <30% flow (severe reduction) signifies tissue is probably irreversibly damaged.

Cerebral blood volume: May be normal or reduced.

■ 80% flow (slightly reduced) referring to oligaemic tissue that will probably survive.

■ <60% flow (moderate reduction) referring to tissue at risk and potentially salvageable by reperfusion.

■ <40% flow (severe reduction) often signifying irreversibly damaged tissue.

Differential diagnosis

Neoplasms and AV malformations may mimic stroke and need to be excluded.

Interventional aspects

The reporting radiologist needs to be aware of the criteria for acute stroke thrombolysis. Currently, 3 h from the time of ictus is generally considered to be the optimal frame for thrombolysis, but the earlier the better. This time may be extended to 6 h if acute imaging reveals potentially salvageable brain tissue.

Acute reporting

■ If the non-contrast examination is normal, proceed to CT perfusion.

- Discuss the options closely with the neuroradiologists and local stroke physicians.

Recommended reading

de Lucas EM, Sánchez E, Gutiérrez A, et al. CT protocol for acute stroke: tips and tricks for general radiologists. *Radiographics* 2008;**28**:1673–87.
Tomandl BF, Klotz E, Handschu R, et al. Comprehensive imaging of ischemic stroke with multisection CT. *Radiographics* 2003;**23**:565–92.

Cerebral venous thrombosis

Summary

Protocol: Non-contrast imaging followed by CT venogram (CTV).

What to look for: Dense asymmetrical veins; subcortical haematoma; infarction; filling defects on CTV.

Report: Describe the affected venous sinus, and secondary effects like haemorrhage or infarction.

Cerebral venous thrombosis can present in numerous ways that can make the diagnosis of early disease difficult. Non-contrast CT is usually the first-line investigation but CTV has proven to have a high sensitivity (up to 95%) for the diagnosis of cerebral venous thrombosis.

Protocol and technique

Contrast enhancement: Non-contrast imaging, followed by CT venography.

CT venography technique: Section thickness 0.625 mm, 100 ml of non-ionic contrast given at 3 ml/s, 45 s prescanning delay, helical acquisitions vertex to C1. Look at source images and multiplanar reformats. Use wide windows to optimally visualize the venous system.

What to look for on CT (Figs 7.12, 7.13)

- In the majority of cases, non-contrast imaging will be completely normal. There are two distinct patterns found in the minority who have an abnormal CT: recently thrombosed vein appearing as the *dense cord sign*; and intravascular blood clot showing as a low density lesion within the vein – the *dense triangle sign*.
- On CTV look for the direct and indirect signs of venous thrombosis.

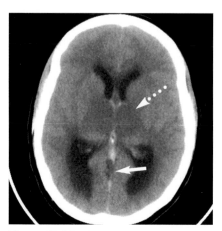 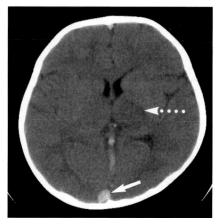

Figure 7.12: Cerebral venous thrombosis. Contrast-enhanced image demonstrates filling defect in the midline internal cerebral vein (arrow). Note the associated bilateral thalamic infarction (dotted arrow) and hydrocephalus.

Figure 7.13: Cerebral venous thrombosis. Non-contrast image demonstrates high density within the inferior sagittal sinus (arrow) and internal cerebral vein, pathognomonic for venous sinus thrombus. Note the early signs of thalamic infarct (dotted arrow).

- Indirect signs include brain oedema, gyral swelling, low-density areas representing venous infarctions with or without haemorrhagic changes.
- The direct evidence for venous thrombosis is a filling defect in a sinus.
- ***Avoid pitfalls:*** Anatomical variations; the right transverse sinus is usually dominant (i.e. larger), the sinuses may be congenitally absent or hypoplastic, prominent arachnoid granulations appear as rounded filling defects.

Acute reporting

- Confirm findings on non-contrast study.
- Evaluate the reformats on CTV and document the location of thrombosis.

Recommended reading

Rodallec MH, Krainik A, Feydy A, et al. Cerebral venous thrombosis and multidetector CT angiography: tips and tricks. *Radiographics* 2006;**26**:S5–S18.

Meningitis

Summary

Protocol: Pre- and post-contrast examination.

What to look for: Prominent CSF spaces; meningeal enhancement; extra-axial collections.

Report: Based on CT findings, meningitis may only be suggested; suggest MRI.

Meningitis is the commonest infection to involve the central nervous system and can be considered in three categories.

- Acute pyogenic (bacterial)
- Lymphocytic (viral).
- Chronic tuberculosis (TB) or fungal infections.

Meningitis is a clinical and microbiological diagnosis. Imaging has a role in monitoring potential complications (about 50% of infected individuals), such as hydrocephalus, empyema and abscess formation, cerebritis, secondary infarction and venous sinus thrombosis.

Protocol and technique

Contrast enhancement: Pre- and post-contrast examination.

Slice collimation: 5 mm or less.

What to look for on CT

- The most common finding in acute meningitis is a normal scan.
- Minor prominence of the ventricles and/or the subarachnoid spaces may be an early sign.
- In more advanced stages, inflammatory exudate fills up the CSF spaces. This may appear quite dense on a non-contrast study.
- Look for abnormal meningeal enhancement on contrast-enhanced images. This is seen in <50% of cases.
- Look carefully for complications: hydrocephalus secondary to plugging of CSF outflow paths by thick inflammatory exudates, abnormal enhancement of ventricular wall suggesting ventriculitis, sterile extra-axial collections, empyema, cerebritis and frank abscesses (abnormally enhancing walls), infarction and venous thrombosis.

Acute reporting

■ Comment on the size of CSF spaces and evidence of any high-density material on the non-contrast study.
■ Describe any complications.

Recommended reading

Jones JN. Inflammatory disease of the brain diagnosed by computed tomography. *J Neurol* 1978;**218**:125–35.

Encephalitis

Summary

Report: Describe the CT findings. Maintain a low threshold to suggest MRI for further evaluation.

Protocol: Non-contrast followed by post-contrast imaging.

What to look for: Low-density changes in temporal lobe, gyriform enhancement.

Encephalitis represents diffuse infection of the brain parenchyma and is commonly caused by viral infections, classically herpes simplex type I (Fig. 7.14). The initial clinical findings may be non-specific, the patient presenting with confusion, headaches and/or seizures. It is therefore important to maintain a low threshold for early imaging. Although CT is inferior to MRI for demonstrating parenchymal inflammation, CT remains the first imaging test usually requested.

Protocol and technique

Contrast enhancement: Pre- and post-contrast imaging.

Slice collimation: 5 mm or less.

What to look for on CT

■ Early scans may be normal.
■ Look for low-density changes within the temporal lobes with or without mass effects. The low-density changes are due to severe parenchymal inflammation (see, for example, Fig. 7.15).

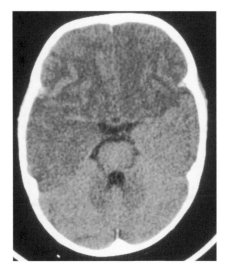

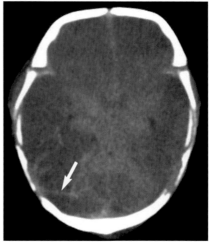

Figure 7.14: Meningoencephalitis.
Low-density changes involving the frontotemporal areas in a young man presenting with confusion. Herpes encephalitis was proven on subsequent lumbar puncture.

Figure 7.15: Meningoencephalitis.
A child with proven meningococcal sepsis and secondary ischaemic changes throughout the brain. Widespread low-density cortical changes are seen along with subtle leptomeningeal enhancement (arrow) on this contrast study.

- Haemorrhagic change within the low-density areas is suggestive of herpes encephalitis.
- On contrast-enhanced images, look for gyriform enhancement.

Differential diagnosis

The initial low-density changes of encephalitis can simulate ischaemia and should be reported in the context of the clinical presentation and distribution of the CT abnormalities.

Acute reporting

Describe the changes seen, but maintain a low threshold to suggest MRI for further evaluation.

Recommended reading

Jones JN. Inflammatory disease of the brain diagnosed by computed tomography. *J Neurol* 1978;**218**:125–35.

Cerebral abscess

Summary

Protocol: Post-contrast imaging.

What to look for: A rim-enhancing lesion(s).

Report: Size, location and number of possible abscesses. Document any secondary effects.

Abscesses develop secondary to pyogenic or fungal infections. CT is the imaging technique of choice to investigate a possible cerebral abscess.

Protocol and technique

Contrast enhancement: Pre- and post-contrast imaging.

Slice collimation: 5 mm or less.

What to look for on CT

■ Cerebritis often heralds the formation of an abscess. It shows up as an ill-defined low-density area in the subcortex and deep white matter. Patchy contrast enhancement may be demonstrated.
■ Established abscesses are seen as smooth-walled rim-enhancing lesions with or without surrounding oedema.
■ Rim enhancement may outlive clinical resolution by many months. Clinical correlation and comparative imaging is therefore essential (Fig. 7.16).

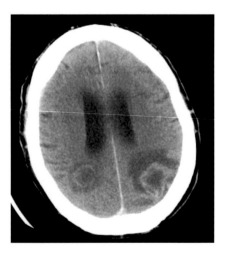

Figure 7.16: Cerebral abscess. Abscesses typically show rim enhancement and are associated with surrounding oedema. This patient, an intravenous drug user, presented with multiple abscesses.

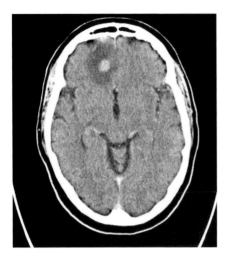

Figure 7.17: Metastases can closely mimic an abscess or a localized haematoma. Clinical correlation and further evaluation with MRI may be necessary to establish the correct diagnosis.

Differential diagnosis

- Malignancies can have similar imaging appearances as abscesses (Fig. 7.17).
- Post-operative changes in the parenchyma can simulate cerebritis.

Acute reporting

- Describe the location and extent of lesions.
- Commenting on any satellite lesions and secondary changes, such as ventriculitis or meningeal involvement (Figs 7.18, 7.19).

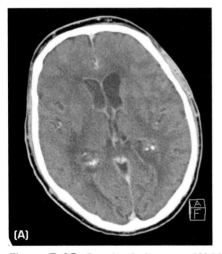
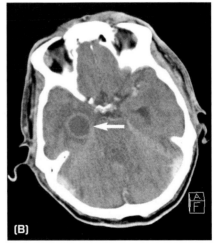

Figure 7.18: Cerebral abscess. (A) Ventriculitis (abnormal ventricular wall enhancement) usually associated with infection. (B) The culprit abscess was located in the right temporal lobe (arrow).

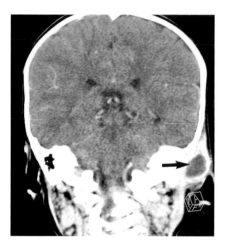

Figure 7.19: Cerebral abscess. When there is clinical evidence of sepsis, a careful evaluation of the extracranial spaces is required. The mastoids (arrow) or middle ear are common sites.

Recommended reading

Stevens EA, Norman D, Kramer RA, Messina AB, Newton TH. Computed tomographic brain scanning in intraparenchymal pyogenic abscesses. *AJR Am J Roentgenol* 1978;**130**:111–4.

Hydrocephalus

Summary

Protocol: Non-contrast examination.

What to look for: Dilated CSF spaces.

Report: Hydrocephalus, level of ventricular compromise, possible aetiology.

Imbalances between CSF production and absorption lead to hydrocephalus, with obstruction to flow rather than increased production being the usual cause. The rate of intracranial pressure rise determines the secondary effects on the brain parenchyma and as such, chronic hydrocephalus in an atrophic brain may not produce the same clinical effects as acute hydrocephalus in a normal brain.

Protocol and technique

Contrast enhancement: Not required for primary diagnosis of hydrocephalus or for comparative imaging. IV contrast will be required when trying to ascertain aetiology.

Slice collimation: 5 mm or less.

What to look for on CT (Fig. 7.20)

- Review any available previous CT.
- If hydrocephalus is present, establish if communicating or non-communicating. 'Communicating hydrocephalus', also known as non-obstructive hydrocephalus, is caused by impaired CSF resorption and may be secondary to haemorrhage, meningitis, Chiari malformation or even the congenital absence of arachnoid granulations. 'Non-communicating or obstructive hydrocephalus', on the other hand, results from an extrinsic compression or an intraventricular mass. Also be aware of unexpected findings, such as a colloid cyst (Fig. 7.21).
- Look for a cause of obstruction: commonly tumours.
- If a shunt is already in situ and the hydrocephalus is worsening, locate the shunt tip to identify any anomalous positioning.
- CT assessment of shunt infection will require contrast administration to look for ventriculitis. Direct CSF examination is more sensitive than imaging.

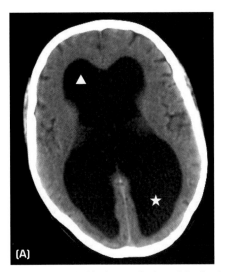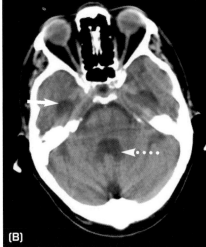

Figure 7.20: Hydrocephalus. Marked prominence of the supratentorial and infratentorial ventricles. Note the **(A)** gross dilatation of the frontal horns (triangle), occipital horns (star) and **(B)** temporal horns (arrow) of the lateral ventricles. The fourth ventricle is also dilated (dotted arrow).

Differential diagnosis

Dilated ventricles (ventriculomegaly) may have other causes such as poor brain development, and clinical correlation is helpful when trying to establish a diagnosis. Ventriculomegaly per se should not be confused

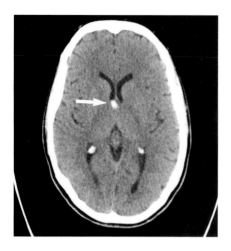

Figure 7.21: Colloid cyst. This is not an obvious hydrocephalus, but is a not-to-be-missed diagnosis of a colloid cyst (arrow). This may be associated with intermittent hydrocephalus and sudden death.

with hydrocephalus. Features that help differentiate between the two conditions include:

- Cortical sulci are typically prominent in ventriculomegaly but are characteristically effaced in hydrocephalus.
- The periventricular regions demonstrate cerebral swelling with interstitial oedema in hydrocephalus, contrasting with typically normal appearances or only small vessel disease in ventriculomegaly.
- A dilated third ventricle displays convex walls with hydrocephalus, and parallel walls with ventriculomegaly.

Acute reporting

- Confirm diagnosis and indicate severity.
- Describe any likely cause.
- Prompt discussion with referring clinician is required.

The post-surgical brain

Summary

Protocol: Non-contrast examination.

What to look for: Normal post-operative changes, hardware, complications.

Report: Bony defect and type, local complications, secondary changes in the remainder of the brain.

The acute post-surgical brain is often imaged when the patient shows unexpected clinical deterioration. Apart from detecting gross pathology such as ischaemia or haemorrhage, the 'normal' appearances of the post-surgical brain should be recognized (Figs 7.22, 7.23).

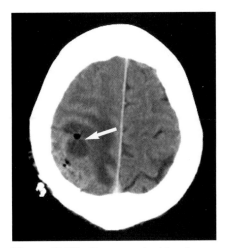 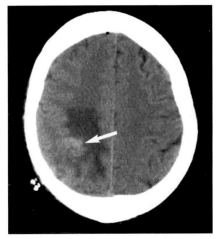

Figure 7.22: Post-surgical brain. Remnant pneumencephalus (arrow) with low-density changes may be a normal post-surgical finding. Serial imaging is required to confirm resolution.

Figure 7.23: Post-surgical brain. High-density focus of haematoma within the operative bed (arrow) is a recognized finding in the immediate post-surgical period. Serial imaging will help resolve any diagnostic difficulty and will be dictated by the patient's clinical status.

Protocol and technique

Contrast enhancement: Usually a non-contrast study is sufficient.

Slice collimation: 5 mm or less; thinner sections may be required through the site of surgery.

What to look for on CT

- First check on bone windows. Has there been a craniotomy or craniectomy? (Figs 7.24, 7.25.)
- Always compare with any available preoperative imaging.
- Mixed density changes in the operative bed may reflect normal post-operative appearances.
- Carefully look for intra- or extra-axial collections. Administer intravenous contrast if in doubt.

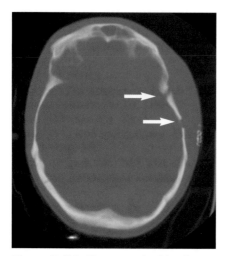

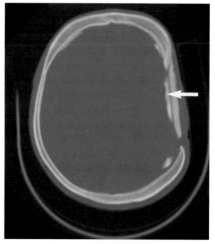

Figure 7.24: Post-surgical brain. Review on bony windows should be the first step in any evaluation of a post-surgical cranial CT as this will usually help clarify the type of operation performed. This patient has had a left-sided craniotomy (arrows).

Figure 7.25: Post-surgical brain. Craniectomy with acrylic cranioplasty with underlying subdural membrane calcification (arrow).

■ Look for areas of abnormal enhancement.
■ Look at the size of the CSF spaces. Is there any evidence of cerebral swelling?
■ Confirm the position of any neurosurgical devices within the brain.

Acute reporting

■ Document any findings that may have resulted from the recent surgery and determine whether these are appropriate or not for the stage of the postoperative recovery.
■ Describe the status of the surrounding parenchyma, CSF spaces and extra-axial space.
■ Describe the position of each catheter and tube and comment if location is satisfactory.

Appendix: Management of acute adverse reactions to iodinated contrast

Management

Management of acute adverse reactions to iodinated contrast

1. Evaluate and maintain ABC.
2. Oxygen 6–10 L.
3. Consider seeking help at any stage (i.e. crash team).
4. Consider transfer to intensive care unit.

Note: most contrast reactions are minor and do not need the above steps.

Urticaria and facial oedema

1. H1-receptor blocker: diphenhydramine PO/IM/IV.
2. If severe or widely disseminated give alpha-agonist: epinephrine SC.

Laryngeal oedema or bronchospasm

1. Give beta-agonist inhalers (bronchiolar dilators, such as salbutamol or metaproterenol 2–3 puffs). Repeat as necessary.
2. Give epinephrine SC, IM or IV, especially if hypotension evident. Repeat in 3–5 min as needed to a maximum of 1 mg.

Pulmonary oedema

1. Give diuretic – furosemide.
2. Consider giving morphine to adults (1–3 mg IV).

Hypotension with tachycardia

1. Elevate legs and keep patient warm.
2. Give IV normal saline or Ringer's lactate.

3. If poorly responsive: epinephrine (1:10 000) slowly IV. Repeat as needed up to a maximum of 1 mg.

Hypotension with bradycardia (vagal reaction)

1. Elevate legs and keep patient warm.
2. Give IV normal saline or Ringer's lactate.
3. IV atropine:

In children: 0.02 mg/kg if patient does not respond quickly to steps 1 and 2. Minimum initial dose of 0.1 mg. Maximum initial dose of 0.5 mg (infant/child), 1.0 mg (adolescent). Atropine dose may be doubled for second administration.

In adults: 0.6–1 mg IV slowly. Repeat atropine up to a total dose of 0.04 mg/kg (2–3 mg) in adult.

Seizures (adults)

Diazepam 5 mg IV.

Medications used to treat adverse reactions to contrast

Medication	Mode of administration	Paediatric dose	Adult dose
Diphenhydramine	PO/IM/IV	1–2 mg/kg, maximum 50 mg	25–50 mg
Epinephrine (1:1000)	SC/IM	0.01 mL/kg (1:1000) maximum 0.3 mL	0.1–0.3 ml (1:1000)
Epinephrine (1:10 000)	IV	0.1 mL/kg, maximum 3 mL/dose	1–3 ml (0.1–0.3 mg)
Atropine	IV	0.02 mg/kg	0.6–1 mg
Furosemide	IV	1–2 mg/kg	20-40 mg

IM = intramuscular; IV = intravenous; SC = subcutaneous; PO = orally.

Recommended reading

The ACR Manual on Contrast Media Version 6, *2008. Available online at: www.acr.org/SecondaryMainMenuCategories/quality_safety/contrast_m anual.aspx*

Index

Page references to *figures, tables and text boxes* are shown in *italics*.